In praise  of Clare Byam-Cook's expert advice

'Whenever I refer patients to Clare I am confident that, if the problem can be solved, she will solve it. Her expertise and calm, confident manner have provided help and reassurance to countless mothers over the years.'

Dr Tim Evans, Royal Physician

'With Mia I had real problems getting her to latch on and was close to giving up when I got advice from Clare. I just can't praise her enough – she has a really straightforward way of describing the latching-on technique.'

Kate Winslet

'As a first-time mum, Clare gave me the confidence to breast-feed successfully and to appreciate that, with the right technique, it can be a totally pain-free and profoundly bonding experience with your baby. It was only because of Clare that I managed to do seven months.'

Trinny Woodall

'This book should be handed out with the first contraction. Clare is a true "baby whisperer" who will save you and your baby hours of torment. Her kind, common-sense and amazingly informed advice was as essential to me as breast-pads and chocolate. Buy this book!'

Kate Beckinsale

'I booked Clare to come round the day my fourth child was born, and the breast-feeding has, for the first time, worked from the first day.'

Emma Freud

'Breast-feeding is one of those things you go through life assuming to be natural and easy, but when I was pregnant I began to hear lots of horror stories about bleeding nipples and awful pain. So I booked Clare to come and see me by way of a pre-emptive strike. It was fantastic. She showed me how to place the baby at the right level using a pillow and pretty early on I was able to feed him, hands-free.'

Helena Bonham Carter

'When I read Clare's book I realised how much I had to learn, and how much could so easily go wrong. The hour or so I spent with her was one of the most valuable in my "motherhood" preparation. I always thought that breast-feeding would be a chore but I have to say it is one of the highlights of my day.'

Gabby Logan

'I have very gratefully accepted Clare's straight-talking, no-nonsense approach . . . Clare's invaluable help has resulted in two happier parents as well.'

Atul J Sabhawal, Consultant Paediatric Surgeon

'Clare really knows what she is talking about.'

Dr John Fysh, Consultant Paediatrician

'It was such a relief to read common-sense advice that was not pompous or judgemental.'

Letter from a breast-feeding GP

'Why isn't your book given to every mum and/or midwife?'

Letter from a client

Top Tips for Breast-feeding

Clare Byam-Cook

Vermilion
LONDON

1 3 5 7 9 10 8 6 4 2

Published in 2008 by Vermilion, an imprint of Ebury Publishing

A Random House Group Company
Copyright © Clare Byam-Cook 2008

Clare Byam-Cook has asserted her right to be identified as the author of this Work in accordance
with the Copyright, Designs and Patents Act 1988

The Random House Group Limited Reg. No. 954009

Addresses for companies within the Random House Group can be found at
www.randomhouse.co.uk

A CIP catalogue record for this book is available from the British Library

The Random House Group Limited supports The Forest Stewardship Council (FSC), the leading international
forest certification organisation. All our titles that are printed on Greenpeace approved FSC certified paper carry
the FSC logo. Our paper procurement policy can be found at www.rbooks.co.uk/environment

Mixed Sources
Product group from well-managed
forests and other controlled sources
www.fsc.org Cert no. TT-COC-2139
© 1996 Forest Stewardship Council

Printed and bound in Great Britain by
Mackays of Chatham plc, Chatham, Kent

ISBN 9780091923464

Copies are a_____ment team

To buy boo_____ks.co.uk

Contents

Acknowledgements

I would like to thank:

Christine and Peter Hill, who have given me the benefit of their wisdom and knowledge on all aspects of caring for mothers and babies – and have also provided many of my clients! Their book *A Perfect Start* is full of sound, practical advice that will both help and reassure anxious new parents, and covers in greater detail many of the subjects mentioned in this book.

Dr John Fysh, Consultant Paediatrician at The Portland Hospital, for taking the time to discuss some of the medical aspects of this book. He also recommends me to his patients, and I am grateful for his support and advice.

Author's Note

I wrote my first book, *What to Expect When You're Breast-feeding ...and What if You Can't?*, to explain how breast-feeding works and what to do if it goes wrong. Breast-feeding is not as easy as everyone makes out (about 50 per cent of mothers give up in the first six weeks) so mothers clearly need more help and advice than they are currently getting. That book covers everything in great detail and is perfect for parents who want to know all the whys and wherefores of breast-feeding, with full instructions and explanations.

However, not every mother wants this much detail and would prefer a smaller and simpler guide to breast-feeding that can be read quickly in a crisis. This book is a bit like the 'quick start' guide that comes with your new TV – it gives you all the information you need to get started and has easy-to-read trouble-shooting sections if things go wrong.

I recommend that you pack this book when you go into hospital so you have it to hand as soon as your baby is born. Many mothers sail through breast-feeding but others struggle and need help very early on. It is also widely acknowledged that many mothers receive a lot of confusing and contradictory advice when they are in hospital and it is hard for them to know whose advice to follow. This book should help you decide.

I hope that everyone who reads this book will succeed at breast-feeding, but if you can't manage it **do not feel a failure.** As you will see in this book, there are genuine reasons why some women can't breast-feed – and formula milk is not liquid poison! The most important thing is that you and your baby are happy and thriving, and that he gets enough milk.

Note: For simplicity and ease of writing, I refer to the baby throughout the book as 'he' and to the father of the baby as 'your husband'. This does not mean that I assume all babies are male and that everyone is married!

1 Preparing for Breast-feeding

There is very little advance preparation needed for breast-feeding other than eating healthily and researching what equipment you will want/need to make feeding go smoothly. Even if you are planning to breast-feed exclusively, I do recommend that you have some bottle-feeding equipment in the house for the following reasons:

- Problems may arise that, temporarily, make breast-feeding difficult (for example, sore nipples, or the baby is unable to latch on).
- Your baby needs to learn to feed from a bottle as well as the breast so he will happily make the transfer if/when you have to stop breast-feeding.
- Very few babies are breast-fed up until the point where they can go straight from breast to beaker.

You will need:

- a box of disposable breast-pads or a minimum of 18 washable ones
- at least three well-fitting maternity bras

- nipple cream (I highly recommend Lansinoh)
- at least one bottle and teat
- a bottle brush
- a steam steriliser, or a small bottle of sterilising fluid or packet of sterilising tablets
- a breast pump (see below and page 124)

You may also need:

- two nipple shields
- two breast shells (if your breasts leak a lot of milk in between feeds)
- a small carton of ready-made formula milk (for use in an emergency only)

Breast pumps
These are an invaluable aid to most mothers. You might need one because:

- you experience primary engorgement (see page 82) and your baby either can't latch on or can't empty your breasts
- you have blocked milk ducts (a pump may help to clear them)
- your nipples are sore and you need some respite
- your baby can't or won't suck efficiently and is therefore not emptying your breasts properly

- you occasionally want to express your milk so someone else can feed your baby
- you want to stimulate milk production if your supply is low
- you have to go back to work but want to carry on giving your baby breast milk

I recommend that you buy, rather than rent, a pump and I also suggest that you invest in an electric rather than a manual pump as these generally work better if you plan to do a lot of expressing. For more on expressing see Chapter 6 'Expressing Milk and Giving Bottles'.

Nipple shields
Nipple shields can be an invaluable aid for many breast-feeding problems and I think it's a great shame that they are not recommended more often. I always use shields made by Medela as they come in both a small and a large size, and I find that the majority of babies suck more effectively when using a smaller shield (most other shields are fairly large). I use them for any of the following issues:

- the baby can't or won't latch on
- the milk flow is too fast
- the baby has a poor sucking action and can't 'milk' the breast efficiently
- when the mother has such sensitive nipples that feeding hurts

even when her baby *is* latched on correctly (this is pretty unusual, but does affect a *small* number of mothers)

See page 76 for more on how to use nipple shields.

Diet during pregnancy

During pregnancy it is important to eat a good, healthy diet and to increase your calorie intake by approximately 200–300 calories a day. You also need to avoid any foods which might be harmful to the baby:

- Any food containing raw eggs because of the risk of salmonella.
- All soft and blue-veined cheese, and any other unpasteurised dairy products. These may contain harmful listeria bacteria.
- Unwashed fruit and vegetables, and raw or under-cooked meat (such as pâté or pork), as these may contain a parasite which can cause Toxoplasmosis.
- All supplements containing vitamin A, and any food (especially liver) with high levels of vitamin A, as large quantities of vitamin A can cause birth defects.

Note: Recent research shows that it is no longer necessary or advisable to avoid peanuts if you have a family history of allergies.

Alcohol

Although it is generally considered safe to drink small amounts of alcohol (between two and four units a week) it is clearly best to drink as little as possible both during pregnancy and when breast-feeding. Binge-drinking is *not* safe and should be avoided at all costs.

Diet when breast-feeding

To give you energy and help maintain a good milk supply, you should eat and drink slightly more than usual and make sure that you are not skipping meals because you are too tired or too busy. You can eat anything you want but some babies get windy and unsettled if you eat garlic, hot spicy foods such as curries, or excessive amounts of citrus fruits. Do drink plenty of fluids.

Drugs and breast-feeding

Most over-the-counter drugs such as paracetamol are safe to take while breast-feeding, but always read the information leaflet to check whether the medication is suitable for breast-feeding mothers. Some drugs (e.g. antibiotics) may give your baby diarrhoea or make him uncomfortable with wind or colic. This should not harm your baby, but if he reacts very badly you should consult your doctor or local pharmacist.

Breast surgery
Some women can breast-feed after breast surgery (e.g. to excise benign or malignant growths, breast enhancement or reduction); others can't. As it is impossible to predict in advance how breast surgery will affect individual women, I would advise all mothers to give breast-feeding a try, but not to feel a failure if they can't do it.

How breast-feeding works
Breasts are designed to produce milk for babies and most breasts work properly and will produce enough milk for your baby. However, some breasts seem to work much better than others and, in my experience, it is mainly down to luck (rather than effort) if you have a good milk supply. Some mothers could easily feed triplets, while others struggle to feed only one. Breast size bears no relation to milk production. (For more on milk and colostrum in the first days after the birth, see page 37.)

Breast milk is produced on a 'supply-and-demand' basis, which means that *your* breasts will react to *your* baby's individual needs: the more he feeds, the more milk they will produce; the less he feeds, the less they will produce. For this reason, it is vital to the success of breast-feeding to allow your baby to feed regularly in order to give the correct messages to your breasts. If you miss feeds and/or give formula top-ups, your breasts will get in a muddle and will almost certainly cut back on production. As long as you feed your baby whenever he is hungry (rather than making him stick to a strict and inflexible feeding schedule – for more on this see page 58), your breasts will normally increase or decrease the amount of milk they are producing to keep in step with his requirements.

The let-down reflex

This is the mechanism that releases the milk from the breasts when your baby feeds and also affects how fast the milk flows. This varies enormously from mother to mother, with some having a very fast let-down, others having a very slow let-down and the majority having a normal or average one. You have no control over your let-down reflex and it is very much the luck of the draw as to how fast or slow it is. But the reason you need to know about it is because this is what dictates how long it will take *your* baby to get enough milk out of *your* breasts. If you have a fast let-down reflex your baby may be able to get all the milk he needs in as little as 10 minutes, whereas a slower let-down may require your baby to take anything from 20 minutes to an hour to feed.

Foremilk and hindmilk

There is a lot of confusion and misunderstanding about the composition of breast milk, with the result that many mothers are given both misleading and incorrect advice on the subject. The general perception seems to be that breasts produce two totally different kinds of milk – the foremilk, which comes out first, and then the hindmilk, which comes right at the end of the feed and will only be reached if the breast is *completely* emptied. With this in mind, mothers are told any of the following:

- You should only use one breast per feed (to ensure that the hindmilk is reached).
- You must completely empty one breast before you swap to the other.
- It will take a baby precisely 20 minutes to reach the hindmilk (or 30 or 40 minutes, depending on the view of the person relaying this information!)

In fact, what actually happens is that the baby starts off with the foremilk, but within a matter of minutes he will be getting the hindmilk. It is therefore totally incorrect to dictate exactly how long a baby needs to feed in order to reach this hindmilk, or to state that a breast must be *completely* empty before the second breast is offered.

One breast or two?
Don't listen to anyone who tells you that you must only use one breast per feed. Instead, see what works best for you. Using only one breast per feed may suit mothers who are producing masses of

milk, but most women find that a single breast does not provide enough milk for their baby. This is what you should do:

- Allow your baby to feed on the first breast for as long as he is sucking properly (see page 20).
- Take him off the breast and wind him (see page 22).
- If he is showing all the signs of being fully fed, you can put him down to sleep.
- If he is still hungry, you should offer him the second breast.
- When he no longer wants to feed on the second breast, you can settle him to sleep.
- Alternate the breast you start on so that each breast gets plenty of stimulation to encourage them to maintain a good milk supply.

After a good feed your baby should settle well and not need feeding again for a reasonable amount of time (roughly three to four hours). If he doesn't do this, he probably needs more milk and you should encourage him to feed a bit longer on one or both of your breasts. When he has had enough milk, he should be contented.

Many mothers only need to use one breast per feed initially, but then find that this stops being enough and they start needing to use both. So do be aware that things can change and you may need to make regular adjustments to the way you feed.

Afterpains

Breast-feeding stimulates the uterus to contract, causing some women to experience cramp-like abdominal pains as they feed. This normally only happens for the first few days after the birth but if they are too intense and painful, it is fine to take a mild painkiller, such as paracetamol.

Note: Always read the information leaflet before taking any medication, to check that it is safe to use when breast-feeding.

2 How to Breast-feed

Some mothers find it very easy to breast-feed, while others struggle right from the outset. Likewise, some babies know instinctively how to latch on and suck correctly, while others need to be taught. Breast shape plays a large part in this – a large breast with flat nipples is much harder for a baby to latch onto than a small breast with protruding nipples. But by using the technique I describe below, most babies can and will latch onto almost any breast.

When breast-feeding goes well it is easy! This is what should happen:

- Your baby wakes up hungry.
- You put him to the breast, he latches on quickly, and **it does not hurt.**
- He sucks slowly and rhythmically until he is full and doesn't want to feed any more.
- He then sleeps soundly (in his crib) until he is hungry and demands another feed (three to four hours later).

- You put him back to the breast and he has another feed. He then goes to sleep once more and the cycle starts all over again.

To achieve this, it helps to get into a good routine:

- Change your baby's nappy before the feed so you don't need to disturb him when he's drowsy and ready to go back to sleep.
- Sit in a comfortable chair with your back well supported.
- Latch your baby on carefully so he is not hurting you.
- Keep feeding him until he won't feed any more – do not stop the second he dozes off.
- Wind him at the end of the feed, even if he is asleep.
- Swaddle him firmly and then put him down in his crib.

If your baby is feeding well he should:

- be contented and sleep well in between feeds
- feed roughly every three to four hours
- have plenty of wet and dirty nappies
- be gaining the right amount of weight

If your baby is not doing this most of the time, you should read the relevant sections in this book to establish what is going wrong (see pages 75 and 97). Don't just assume that you have a 'difficult' baby who needs endless feeding and cuddling.

Latching on

I recommend using pillows to begin with, as they will support your baby and make you more comfortable and relaxed. I prefer ordinary bed pillows rather than special feeding pillows, as they fit closer to your body and give your baby better support. At each feed you should:

● Sit comfortably and arrange your pillows to the correct height.

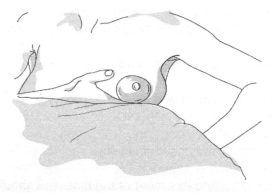

Lifting the breast

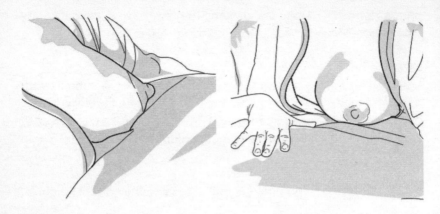

Placing the breast on a pillow
(side view)

Placing the breast on a pillow
(front view)

- Lay your baby on his side on the top pillow, with his tummy close to your body and his mouth (not his nose) directly in front of your nipple Do not lean forward to your baby – instead bring him to you.
- Hold him firmly (but not roughly) so that you have good control of his head.
- Brush your nipple against his lips to stimulate him to open his mouth – if he is crying you don't need to do this as his mouth will already be wide open!

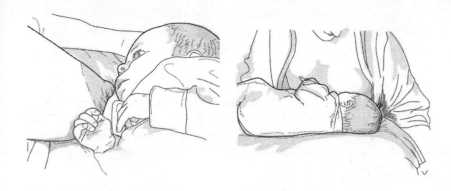

Baby lying with mouth directly in front of nipple

Lying your baby on his side (front view)

- Move him swiftly to your breast so that you get as much nipple as possible into his mouth before he closes it.
- The first few sucks will feel surprisingly strong, but he should soon settle into slow rhythmic sucking that doesn't hurt at all.
- Relax your shoulders and let him carry on feeding.

Don't worry if it takes several attempts to latch your baby on – this is normal. But if he can't manage at all (maybe because you have very large, flat or inverted nipples), you need to help him by shaping your breast so that it fits better into his mouth. This is like trying to post a large parcel into a small letterbox – if the opening is too narrow you have to squash the parcel to make it fit in!

How to shape your breast
- Lift your breast and place it on a pillow (see pages 13 and 14).
- Lay your baby on his side on the top pillow, with his tummy close to your body and his mouth (not his nose) directly in front of your nipple. Do not lean forward to your baby – instead bring him to you (see page 15).
- 'Shape' your breast, using the hand which is on the same side as the breast your baby is about to feed from.
- Slide your hand underneath your breast and place the balls of your thumb and third finger level with your nipple and on the outside of your areola at the 3 o'clock and 9 o'clock position.
- Gently squeeze your breast until your nipple protrudes – if you squeeze too hard your nipple may invert.

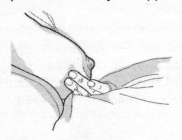 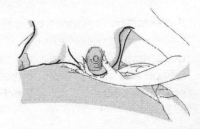

- Place your hand under your baby's head and shoulders so that you have good control of his head.
- Brush your nipple against his lips and, as soon as he opens his mouth, move him swiftly to your breast so that you get as much nipple and areola as possible into his mouth before he closes it. I describe this procedure as 'shape and shove'!
- If your baby closes his mouth on the wrong bit of your nipple, or misses it completely, check that your nipple is going above (not under) his tongue and that your nipple is level with his mouth. Babies often lunge upwards towards the breast, so if he keeps missing, try bringing him to the breast from below the nipple.
- Once your baby is latched on, you can *gradually* let go of your breast and remove your hand – but don't let go too quickly, or he may be pushed off as your breast flattens out again. You may need to plump up the pillow where your hand squashed it down.
- If he comes off when you let go of your breast, go back to square one, and release your breast more slowly the next time.

If you still can't get him on, ask your husband to help – men tend to be very practical and he may be able to see if you are not getting it quite right! If your baby can't latch on at all, even when using the 'shape and shove' method, you will need to experiment with nipple shields, expressing etc. (See 'Baby can't latch on', page 75.)

The 'nose to nipple' theory

I find it extraordinary that mothers are told to hold their baby 'nose to nipple' rather than 'mouth to nipple', and I think this advice actually makes it harder for a baby to latch on quickly and painlessly. Mothers are told to brush their nipple against the baby's nose and then wait until his mouth 'gapes wide open' before allowing him to latch on. I am totally against this advice for the following reasons:

- Many babies don't know that they must open their mouth really wide and these babies become very agitated and upset if they are made to wait until they do.
- Some babies physically *can't* open their mouth wide enough to latch onto a large breast.
- Lining your baby up with his nose (rather than his mouth) in front of your nipple makes it much harder for him to latch on.
- If he does manage to latch on, he has to pull your nipple away from his nose towards his mouth and this pulling creates sore nipples.
- Bending the nipple slows the milk flow so feeds last longer.
- Your breast may empty unevenly and this can cause mastitis.

Whenever I see a client who has been taught this method, I can quickly demonstrate that 'mouth to nipple' works better. I also point out that if she was bottle-feeding her baby, she would never dream of irritating him by flicking the teat against his nose and then refusing to put it in his mouth until she deems that he has opened it wide enough! So why do this to a breast-fed baby?

Note: Don't worry if you *have* been using the 'nose to nipple' method – your baby will be happy to change to a different technique if it makes it easier for him to latch on.

Is my baby feeding effectively?

The next step is to check that your baby is latched on correctly, is sucking well and is also getting enough milk. Without doing this, you can quickly end up with sore nipples and/or a dehydrated, hungry and unsettled baby. **Sucking on the breast for hours on end does not mean he is getting plenty of milk!**

Step one: Is your baby latched on correctly?

- He should have all the nipple and most of the areola in his mouth so that his gums are well behind the base of your nipple.
- His mouth should be wide open and his lips curled back.
- His nose and chin should be gently pressed against your breast. You don't need to press your breast away from his nose – if you hold him so close that he can't breathe, he will let go of your nipple.
- His head should not be curled in or extended too far back – he should be coming at a right angle to the breast.

- He should have his mouth (not his nose) directly in front of your nipple.
- His sucking should not hurt at all.
- If your baby is on at slightly the wrong angle, you will see your breast being pulled towards his mouth. Move him towards the direction of the pull while he continues to suck – when he is in the right place, the pulling will stop.

Note: Always use your finger to release the suction before removing your baby from the breast. Do not lick your finger before you put it in his mouth – this is unhygienic and unnecessary.

Step two: Is he sucking correctly?
If your baby is not sucking properly he may get no more milk out of your breast than he would get if he was sucking on a dummy. It is therefore vital to know the difference between effective and ineffective feeding.

When sucking well:

- He will start off with fairly short quick sucks and then, once the milk starts to flow, his sucks will become slower, deeper and more rhythmic in action.
- The top and bottom of his jaw will be moving and this movement will extend right up the jaw-line as far as his ears.
- He will feed fairly continuously for a good 10 minutes or so without you needing to stroke his cheek or tickle his feet to keep him going.

Signs of poor sucking are:

- pursed lips and hollowed cheeks
- small, infrequent and shallow sucks
- falling asleep at the breast well before he has had enough milk

Step three: How will I know when my baby has had enough milk?
This would be easy if breasts worked like a gasometer and visibly deflated with each ounce of milk that the baby extracts! Unfortunately this doesn't happen, so it is only through experience that you will learn to judge whether your baby has stopped feeding because he is full or whether he has dozed off too soon.

Tips to bear in mind include:

- At the start of each feed your breasts will feel firm and full.
- As they empty, your breasts will feel softer and less full.
- When your baby first latches on he will usually suck strongly and continuously with very few pauses.
- As his tummy fills up with milk, his sucking will slow down and he will pause more.
- When he won't feed any more on either breast, he is probably full and you can put him down to sleep.

Now you have to wait and see what happens! If he lasts three to four hours before he wants to feed again he almost certainly got enough milk. But if he wants to feed again much sooner than this, he clearly fell asleep too soon and you should try to keep him feeding for a bit longer at the next feed.

When he has had enough milk he should:

- settle well in his crib
- sleep well between feeds
- pass plenty of urine
- gain the right amount of weight

Step four: How long should the feed last?

The answer is: long enough for your baby to get enough milk to last him until the next feed, which, ideally, would be about three to four hours later. The duration of your feeds will depend on how strongly your baby sucks, how well he is latched on, how fast your milk flows (see 'The let-down reflex', page 7) and also how much milk you have. An average-length feed would last approximately 20 minutes, a slow feed can take anything up to an hour, and a fast feed can be over in 10 minutes or less.

Winding

There is a myth that breast-fed babies don't need winding, but I'm afraid that this is certainly not true – a breast-fed baby will often need just as much winding as a bottle-fed baby, especially if he is badly attached to the breast. You should always wind a baby at the end of a feed and also at any point during a feed when he seems uncomfortable.

- The best way to wind a baby is to hold his body firmly against your chest with one hand, while using the other hand to push gently into the small of his back.
- When a baby has wind, his back will usually curve outwards and his spine will resist your efforts to straighten it.
- If a baby has little or no wind, his spine will feel very flexible.
- Your baby may bring up a small amount of milk when he burps – this is called 'possetting' and is absolutely normal.

Hiccups

It is very common for a baby to have hiccups. Most babies are untroubled by them and will happily carry on with whatever they are doing – feeding, sleeping etc. But if your baby *is* unsettled with hiccups, you could try offering him some cool boiled water (either from a bottle or from a spoon) to see if this helps.

Winding: holding baby against chest

Settling your baby after feeds

Some babies settle quickly and easily after feeds, others are much slower, and some babies find it almost impossible to go to sleep without help from you. You won't know what type of baby you have until you start trying to settle him. The most important factor is to be clear in your own mind that sleep is the one and only thing he needs so that you can concentrate on getting him to sleep rather than worrying whether he needs more feeding or winding.

To achieve this you should:

- feed your baby for as long as he is sucking properly
- change his nappy if it's dirty (or you didn't change it at the start of the feed)
- wind him thoroughly
- swaddle him so that he feels secure

A baby will normally sleep longer and better when swaddled, so ask a midwife, relative or friend to show you how to do this. Most babies feel secure with their whole body firmly swaddled, but if your baby clearly hates having his arms confined and/or he wants to suck his thumb, you can wrap him up leaving his arms free.

Don't risk overheating your baby (use a cotton sheet and fewer clothes and blankets in hot weather) and always put him down to sleep on his back or his side but *not* on his tummy. (For more information on this, see 'Cot death', page 43.)

- He may fall asleep immediately or he may gaze around for a bit before dozing off. Either is fine!
- If he starts grizzling or crying *gently*, leave him for a while to see whether he settles – it's not unkind to do this as many babies will only fall asleep if they are left to cry. If you keep picking up a crying baby you may end up making him thoroughly overtired and even more incapable of going to sleep.
- If he is still awake after about 10 minutes but his crying is at the same level or diminishing, you can leave him for a little bit longer. You could also offer him a dummy, rock his crib and/or gently pat his back.
- If his crying escalates and he is clearly becoming more unsettled, you should pick him up to wind him again and calm him down. If absolutely nothing (i.e. winding, rocking or dummy) settles him, you need to return to square one and put him back on the breast. If he still won't settle, you may need to offer him a top-up bottle (see page 72).

Most babies will fall asleep fairly quickly but if your baby is *always* really hard to settle you should consult your health visitor or GP. If he is suffering from a problem such as colic or reflux he needs a proper diagnosis and medical treatment. Cranial osteopathy (see page 117) and altering your diet (if you think your baby is reacting badly to food you are eating) may also help.

Dummies

Opinion is divided on the use of dummies. In general they are frowned upon, as prolonged and excessive use is thought to have an adverse effect on a child's speech and intelligence, but conversely, more recent research suggests that using a dummy reduces cot deaths. Personally, I loathe them, but, nonetheless, they can be invaluable in settling some babies.

Here are my tips:

- Do not use a dummy on a baby who can't go to sleep because he is still hungry.
- Only use a dummy if you cannot settle your baby without one. Don't automatically put it in his mouth every time you put him down to sleep – wait and see if he can settle without it.
- Don't use it just to stop your baby crying (for example, when you are changing his nappy).
- Don't use a dummy when you are walking your baby in a pram or buggy, as the movement should be enough to rock him to sleep.

If you follow these guidelines, your baby is unlikely to become addicted to the dummy and will usually stop using it of his own accord once he no longer needs it. This normally happens at about three months when a baby either stops needing something to suck on before going to sleep, or he discovers his thumb and uses that instead.

Note: Dummies need to be washed and sterilised frequently. Putting the dummy in your own mouth and sucking on it does not make it germ-free and safe to go back in your baby's mouth. This particularly applies if you have a cold or any other infection, which may then be transmitted to your baby.

Different feeding positions
Although I recommend that mothers begin by using pillows when feeding, there are other positions you may prefer (or need) to use.

Cradling in your arm
This is the easiest way to feed when you are out and about with your baby. Your baby's head should lie halfway down your arm (see overleaf) and should not be cradled in the crook of your arm – this will tilt his head the wrong way and make it difficult for him to latch on easily. You can also place a pillow or small cushion under your arm to support the weight of your baby and encourage you to relax your shoulders.

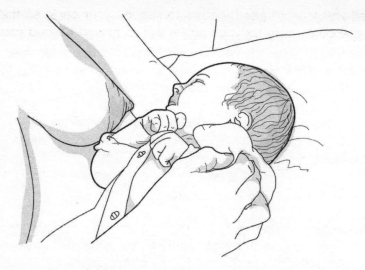

Cradling him halfway down your arm

The football hold

This is the ideal way to feed twins simultaneously but it is not so good for feeding a single baby, especially if he is large. This is because you have to tuck your baby under your arm (see opposite) and it is very hard to do this without him being pushed out of position when his feet touch the surface you are leaning against (e.g. the back of the chair). The football hold only works well if you position yourself well forward (using pillows to support your back) so that there is enough room for your baby's feet to extend beyond your back.

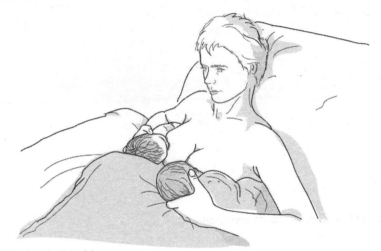

The football hold

However, I do occasionally use the football hold when I come across a baby who feeds perfectly well on one breast but refuses point-blank to feed on the other. As far as I can judge, the baby seems to have developed a phobia for that particular breast, but can be fooled into feeding on it if you use the football hold. This baby will usually happily revert to feeding normally on that breast after only five minutes or so of using this hold. But if your baby continues to reject the same breast whenever you try to feed him without using the football hold, it might be worth consulting a cranial osteopath to see whether there is a physical reason why he cannot feed normally on that side.

Note: I don't recommend using the football hold to deal with problems such as sore nipples or blocked milk ducts as I think these issues can (and should) be resolved by correct latching.

Lying down

I am not a great advocate of this way of feeding for the following reasons:

- It increases the risk of cot death (see page 43).
- It can be difficult to latch your baby on correctly.
- It is likely that both you and your baby will fall asleep, so when you wake up you will have no idea how well or for how long your baby has fed.
- If your baby regularly falls asleep before he has taken a full feed, your breasts will be under-stimulated and may start producing less milk. Your baby might also find it hard to catch up on his milk intake later on in the day.

- If a baby gets used to falling asleep cuddling up to his mother, he may find it hard to settle when put to sleep elsewhere (e.g. in a Moses basket). This can lead to long-term sleep problems.

If, however, a mother can't sit up (because she has really painful stitches or haemorrhoids), she may need to feed lying down for a few days. Try experimenting with different positions to see which works best for you and your baby.

Feeding twins

If your twins are strong and healthy and you have plenty of milk, breast-feeding twins is easier than bottle-feeding. But if your twins are premature or small and/or you don't have enough milk, you may need to combine breast-feeding with top-up bottles until they get stronger or your supply improves.

- Start by feeding each baby separately.
- If they both feed well, you can then try to feed them simultaneously using the 'football hold' (see page 29).
- The babies can remain on the same breast throughout the feed.
- Alternate the breast each baby has at subsequent feeds (as one twin may be better at emptying the breast than the other).
- Offer a top-up after feeds if your milk supply is low and/or your babies are not feeding or settling well (see page 72).

- Whenever you give a top-up, you should express after the feed to take off any milk that is left behind and/or to stimulate your supply.
- If you cannot produce enough milk, don't feel a failure if you have to supplement with formula.

Hygiene

It is important to be meticulous about hygiene as it is easy to spread germs between two babies. You don't need to wash your hands in between handling one baby and the other during feed times, but you should wash your hands after nappy changes, before preparing bottles etc., just as you would if you only had one baby.

- The babies can suck on the same breast (without you needing to wash it) but they should not suck from the same bottle or share a dummy. Using different-coloured rings on the bottles will help avoid confusion.
- If one baby has an infection (e.g. thrush in his mouth) you must wash and sterilise everything very thoroughly and you should also wash your hands carefully every time you handle that baby.
- If either baby develops an infection or a minor illness such as a cold, you should keep them apart until the ill one is better.

Most twins like to be physically close to each other and will usually settle better if they are put to sleep in the same cot. But if one twin keeps being disturbed and woken by the other, it is better to separate them than to have two wakeful babies!

3 The First Few Days

These first days are probably the most important in terms of establishing breast-feeding. If you get your feeding technique right at this stage, breast-feeding should go smoothly and you are less likely to develop any problems. Unfortunately this is also a time when things can go wrong and mothers are subjected to a lot of conflicting advice, which leaves them confused and stressed. In this chapter I look at the various problems that a mother might encounter, and give firm advice as to what to do.

The first 24 hours

Ideally, you would feed your baby within an hour of his birth (because this is when his sucking reflex is at its strongest), and a midwife will normally help you do this. But if your baby doesn't want to feed or if you are too tired after a long labour, it is perfectly all right to wait until you get to the post-natal ward. Some babies are very hungry and wakeful after the birth and start feeding immediately, while others are very sleepy and may not want to feed much at first. You need not worry if:

- your baby latches on and feeds well, but only has about three feeds in the first 24 hours
- he sleeps soundly for the first 12 hours, but then wakes and feeds well from then on

You should take action if he:

- has still not had a good feed after 12 hours
- is crying and trying to feed but is unable to latch onto your breast
- feeds endlessly but then cries every time you try to settle him in his cot
- only does a few sucks at the breast and then falls asleep
- stops waking for feeds
- is not passing urine

This baby is clearly not getting enough milk and will quickly become dehydrated if he is not fed soon.

This is what you should do:

- Shape your breast (see page 16) to help him latch on.
- If he still can't latch on and/or feed efficiently, try to hand-express some colostrum (see below) and feed it to him with a syringe.

- If you don't have enough colostrum you should offer him some formula, preferably using a bottle (see 'Nipple/teat confusion', page 51).
- Make sure he continues to be fed (by breast or bottle) at least four-hourly and put a tissue in his nappy so that you can see whether he is passing urine.

Babies who are getting enough milk go to sleep after a feed (without the need to be cuddled to stop them crying) and they pass urine regularly.

Colostrum

Towards the end of pregnancy your breasts will start producing colostrum and this is the milk that your baby will have for the first three or four days before your full milk comes in. Colostrum is more like cream than milk, so your baby only needs a small amount at each feed – far less than he would need if he was being fed with formula milk.

It is important to be aware of the following:

- It is harder for a baby to extract colostrum than to extract milk, so correct latching at every feed is particularly important.

- There is not much colostrum in your breasts, so you should expect feeds to be relatively short – ideally lasting less than half an hour.
- If your baby wants to feed for a great deal longer than this, he may be latched on incorrectly and therefore not able to get the colostrum as quickly and easily as he should.
- If your baby is having long feeds (because he is latched on badly) you will almost certainly develop sore nipples.
- A baby that has fed well will usually stop feeding of his own accord and will settle well when you put him back in his cot.
- If your baby does not settle well after a feed, he is almost certainly still hungry.
- You should use both breasts at each feed, as there is no such thing as fore and hind colostrum.
- A small number of women do not have enough colostrum and need to supplement with formula until the milk comes in. Don't worry if you need to do this – giving formula at this stage will have no detrimental effect on long-term breast-feeding. Your milk *will* still come in and your baby *won't* lose his ability to suck on the breast. (See 'Nipple/teat confusion', page 51.)

If your baby is latching on correctly and feeding well, you should be able to 'feed on demand' (see page 55) as he will give you clear signs as to when he needs feeding and when he has finished feeding. You would expect him to cry when he's hungry, feed reasonably quickly and then fall into a contented sleep when he's had enough. If he has taken a good feed, he should also last at least one hour (but preferably two to three hours) before he asks to be fed again.

But if your baby is feeding a lot longer and more frequently than this he is clearly not getting enough colostrum. Keep checking your latching technique and give formula if necessary.

When your milk comes in

Your full milk usually comes in around three to four days after the birth; but it will sometimes arrive as early as day two, or to be delayed for a week or more. When your milk is in, your breasts will feel firmer and a lot fuller and the colour of the milk will change from the yellowish consistency of colostrum to a watery milky colour. Some mothers will have so much milk that they become engorged (see page 82) while others barely notice their milk is in.

Frequency of feeds

As soon as your milk comes in it is essential that your breasts are emptied regularly throughout the day and night in order to keep the supply going. You would normally expect your baby to feed at least every three to four hours, thus having anything from six to nine feeds a day. If he regularly takes more than nine feeds a day you should try to get him to take bigger feeds so that he needs feeding less often.

- Try not to feed your baby more frequently than every two hours (timed from the start of one feed to the start of the next).
- Feed him at least every four hours during the day, even if it means waking him. If you feed him less frequently than this, he will almost certainly feed a lot more during the night to make up for his low milk intake during the day.
- Your baby can go longer than four hours at night provided he has fed regularly during the day and his weight is fine.

Note: If you are advised to feed your baby more frequently for medical reasons (if he is jaundiced, for example) you should, of course, follow that advice.

Don't miss any feeds
While you are trying to establish and maintain a good milk supply, it is not a good idea to miss out any feeds (for instance, in the middle of the night) because this will confuse your breasts and may reduce your milk supply. If you are absolutely exhausted, you could occasionally substitute a night-time breast-feed with a bottle but the more you do this the more detrimental it will be to your milk supply.

Expressing
When your milk first comes in, you might have considerably more than your baby needs. It is fine to express some of the surplus milk

to keep in the freezer for future use, but don't express so much that you over-stimulate your breasts. You might also express at this stage if your baby is very sleepy (maybe because he is jaundiced), and is taking less milk than he needs. By expressing, you will maintain a good supply of milk, and you can also top him up with your expressed milk if he is too sleepy to feed properly from the breast. For more on expressing, see Chapter 6 'Expressing Milk and Giving Bottles'.

4 Coming Home from Hospital

Arriving home with a new baby can be daunting as well as exciting. Ideally you would have someone (such as your husband or mother) to stay with you for the first two weeks or so, until you have got used to the responsibility of caring for your baby on your own. During this time you should:

- rest as much as possible
- keep visitors to a minimum
- share the care of your baby – you don't have to do everything to be a good mother!

Cot death
I hate to raise the subject of cot death but, as I realise that many parents start worrying about this almost as soon as they arrive home with their precious baby, I think this is a good time to discuss safety issues.

The incidence of cot death dropped dramatically with the 'back to sleep' campaign and the following guidelines provide additional information to help keep your baby safe. It is currently recommended that:

- The safest place for a baby to sleep is in a cot in the parents' bedroom for the first six months.
- A baby is laid on his back to sleep, not on his tummy.
- Your baby's head is left uncovered in his cot. You should lie him down with his feet touching the end of the cot – to prevent him slipping under the blankets.
- You do not let anyone smoke near your baby. (Parents who smoke anywhere in the house put their baby at a greater risk than non-smokers.)
- You should not let your baby get too hot.
- You should not let your baby sleep in bed with you, especially if you smoke, have been drinking alcohol or taking medications that make you sleepy.
- You should not feed your baby in bed if you are so tired that you might fall asleep.
- You should not sleep with your baby on a sofa or armchair.

If you can follow all the above suggestions, your baby will be receiving the best possible care and you should therefore try not to become too anxious about anything untoward happening to him.

Where should my baby sleep?
There are many different views as to where a baby should sleep in the first few weeks. Although research (as mentioned above) has shown that it is best to put a baby to sleep in a separate cot, some childcare experts continue to disagree with this and think that co-sleeping with your baby is an important part of mother–baby bonding, that it promotes breast-feeding and that it is safe. They say that a baby needs to remain close to his mother in order to feel secure and loved, and that it is wrong to deprive him of this comfort.

I completely disagree! **I think every mother needs to appreciate that a normal healthy baby, whose needs have been met, will sleep soundly and happily wherever you put him.**

Although, for safety reasons, it is best for the baby to sleep in your bedroom, this may not suit all parents for a number of reasons:

- A small bedroom may not have enough space for a cot.
- If you are a light sleeper, having your baby in your bedroom is likely to disturb your sleep unnecessarily, as you will wake with all his little baby noises rather than only being woken when he actually needs attention.
- If you are a noisy sleeper, you might find that you are waking your baby, rather than him waking you!
- Having your baby in your bedroom will result in both you *and* your husband being woken at feed times. This is fine if your husband

wants to be fully involved, but if he has to go to work in the morning it seems a bit unnecessary to have both of you suffering from a lack of sleep. You at least should be able to catch up on lost sleep with a daytime nap.

If you want or need to put your baby in a separate room at night, make sure he is within earshot – use a baby monitor if he is too far away for you to hear him easily.

During the day, your baby can sleep anywhere that suits you, providing you can see or hear him. Young babies don't need quiet or darkness to keep them asleep and it may also help them to distinguish between night and day if they are only put to sleep in a bedroom at night. However, once you notice that your baby *is* becoming sensitive to noise, you will probably find that he will sleep longer and better during his daytime naps if you put him to sleep in his bedroom with the curtains drawn. This usually happens after about three months.

Note: Babies tend to sleep longer and better when they are lying flat (in a Moses basket, pram etc.) than they do when sitting up in a baby seat.

Room temperature

When you take your baby home your house will need to be warmer than usual but not as hot as it was in hospital. A house temperature of about 18–20°C will be warm enough for your baby – you can keep your house cooler than this, but it might seem rather chilly when you are breast-feeding, changing his nappy, bathing him etc. Your baby will come to no harm if he is slightly too warm or slightly too cold; he is only at risk if you get it so completely wrong that he gets far too hot or freezing cold.

During the winter months you will need to make sure that his room does not get too cold at night when the central heating goes off – cold is a common cause of a baby waking at night, especially as he gets older and starts wriggling out from under his blankets. The most economical way to keep your baby's room warm is to use a convector heater or an electric radiator with thermostatic controls, and he may need to start wearing a warm sleepsuit or sleeping bag.

Note: Whenever I come across a particularly anxious mother, who worries obsessively about whether her house is too warm or too cold, I ask her this question: Are you ever planning to take your baby out of your house, and if so, will you only venture forth if the temperature outside is exactly the same as it is indoors? Common sense and suitable clothing are all that you need!

Midwives and health visitors
Your community midwife will normally visit you shortly after you get home (the hospital arranges this) and will give you her contact number. She will continue to visit you regularly until your baby is

about 10 days old. If you are worried about your own or baby's health, don't be afraid to ring your midwife or GP, or even to go to your local Accident and Emergency unit.

The health visitor will usually call by on or around day 10. She will give you a booklet in which to keep records of your baby's development, weight etc. She will also tell you where your nearest baby clinic is and how to get hold of her should you need to.

Dehydration

Within the first week or so of birth, a baby can become dehydrated very quickly if he is not getting enough milk on a regular basis. This rarely happens when a baby is being bottle-fed (as it is pretty obvious if he is not feeding well), but is far less easy to spot when a baby is breast-feeding. I regularly see babies who are dehydrated (some of whom need to go back into hospital) and many of their parents were totally unaware that anything was wrong – mainly because they had been assured by the midwives that their baby was feeding well.

To avoid this happening to you, please be aware of the following:

- Your baby will only get milk out of your breasts if he is latched on correctly and is sucking properly.
- Not all mothers have enough colostrum and/or milk to give their baby – even if he is sucking well.

- The reason why midwives and health visitors wrongly reassure mothers that all is well is that many of them believe that every baby who is breast-feeding is automatically getting plenty of milk. This is based on the mistaken assumption that *all* babies feed perfectly and that *all* mothers have plenty of milk. So please do **not** be reassured that all is well if your baby is showing classic signs of dehydration (see overleaf).
- Don't be misled into thinking that your baby wouldn't sleep well if he was hungry and needed feeding; although most babies will cry if they are hungry and won't settle back to sleep until they have had enough milk, others can become drowsy and lethargic and stop waking for feeds.

Your baby is breast-feeding well if he:

- is waking regularly for feeds – approximately every three to four hours
- settles well after feeds – i.e. goes to sleep in his *own* bed
- is producing at least six wet nappies a day
- does not lose more than 10 per cent of his birth weight
- starts regaining weight after about day four

Your baby is *not* breast-feeding well (and may be becoming dehydrated) if he:

- keeps crying for a feed but then falls asleep after only a few sucks at the breast
- becomes sleepy and listless and stops waking for feeds
- is not passing much urine
- is feeding for hours on end but never seems satisfied
- wakes and starts crying every time you try to settle him in his own bed
- only stops crying when you cuddle him and/or take him into bed with you

Your baby *is* dehydrated if:

- he goes more than six hours without passing urine (putting a tissue in his nappy will make this easier to check)
- his urine is concentrated and smelly
- his mouth and lips are dry
- tiny orange or pink crystals (urates) appear in his nappy
- he is very drowsy and hard to wake
- he has a sunken fontanelle (the soft bit at the top of his skull where the bones have not yet fused)

When a baby is dehydrated, it is important to get more milk into him as soon as possible. You should do this with a bottle (*not* your breast), giving him your own milk if you can express enough, and using formula if you can't. In most cases, one or two bottle-feeds will be enough to raise a baby's energy levels and enable him to feed properly from the breast later on in the day. If this happens you should, of course, stop bottle-feeding him and settle into a normal breast-feeding pattern.

If you can't get your baby to drink at least 30 ml (1 oz) of milk he may need to be admitted to hospital to be fed by tube or intravenous infusion. If in doubt, do not delay ringing your hospital for advice – even in the middle of the night.

Nipple/teat confusion

If a baby can't latch on and/or needs to be given extra milk, many hospitals will insist that the baby is fed with a cup rather than a bottle to avoid 'nipple/teat confusion'. The mother is told that even one bottle of milk will ruin breast-feeding for ever by causing the baby to lose his ability to suck on the breast. This is complete nonsense! I regularly see babies who have been fed by bottle for days or even weeks and most of them can go straight to the breast as soon as they are given the right help (i.e. by shaping the breast, see page 16). While cup-feeding in hospital is fine for a couple of feeds, once you are home I think you should use a bottle, for the following reasons:

- Cup-feeding requires the skill of an experienced midwife to ensure that the milk goes down the baby's throat (rather than his clothes!) and a new mother is unlikely to be this skilled.
- When cup-feeding it is hard to see exactly how much milk your baby is drinking or to judge how much he wants, so he may end up getting less milk than he needs.
- There is no evidence to suggest that giving a few bottle-feeds will confuse a breast-fed baby.
- If a baby is given a bottle because he can't or won't suck on the breast, it seems illogical to blame the bottle if the problem continues.
- I take the view that sucking on a bottle is better than no sucking at all – because lapping milk from a cup requires no effort by your baby.
- If your baby is weak or premature, it is better to check whether he is able to suck from anything (i.e. a bottle) before wasting his energy trying to get him to suck on the breast.

5 Settling into a Feeding Routine

Even when breast-feeding is going really well, many mothers still worry about whether they are doing everything right. Unfortunately, it is common for a mother to find that everyone tells her something different and it can be hard to know whose advice to follow. This chapter covers all the questions that I have been asked over the years and, where appropriate, gives the different views that might be expressed.

Weight gain
Monitoring your baby's weight is very important as this is the best indication as to whether he is getting enough food and is developing as he should.

- It is normal for a baby to lose up to 10 per cent of his birth weight in the first four days.
- If he loses much more than this you **must** offer him more milk, using a bottle if necessary.

- After day four, he should start gaining weight and be back to his birth weight by days 10–14.
- From then on his weight gain should roughly follow the centile chart in your Child Health Record booklet.
- If your baby's weight is falling *well* below the curve on his chart, you should consult a doctor.

How much milk does my baby need?

When breast-feeding it is still useful to know roughly how much milk your baby should be having so that you can work out how much to express for full feeds, top-ups etc.

Babies under the age of four months need approximately 150 ml (5 oz) of milk per kg of body weight (or 2½–3 oz per lb), during each 24-hour period.

Metric

For a 3 kg baby on six feeds a day, you would multiply 3 kg by 150 ml = 450 ml. Divided by six feeds = 75 ml per feed.

Imperial

For a 7 lb baby on seven feeds a day, you should multiply 7 lb by 3 oz = 21 oz. Divided by seven feeds = 3 oz per feed.

Babies rarely take exactly the same amount at each feed, so don't worry if the amount he wants varies by as much as 30 ml (1 oz) or more. As this is only a rough guide, it doesn't matter if your baby regularly takes slightly more or less than this – as long as his weight gain is good, you will be getting it right.

Does my baby need extra water?
Neither a breast-fed nor a bottle-fed baby should need any extra water as milk provides all the fluids he requires. But you might occasionally want to offer some cool, boiled water if:

- the weather is particularly hot and your baby appears thirsty rather than hungry
- your baby is unsettled in between feeds
- your baby is constipated

Do be careful not to give so much water that your baby is then too full to take his milk feed. There are no calories in water, so you shouldn't give him water if he is hungry or if his weight gain is poor.

Feeding on demand
Feeding on demand means being flexible on feed times rather than insisting the baby conforms to a really strict routine. It does *not* mean you should feed your baby every time he cries, nor does it

mean you should have no routine at all. Babies cry for all sorts of reasons and it is important to find out *why* he is crying, rather than automatically assuming that he is hungry and needs another feed. Babies are like toddlers – they thrive on regular meals and sleep times.

When breast-feeding is going really well, most babies need to feed approximately once every three to four hours. If your baby *regularly* needs to feed *much* more frequently than this, it is likely to be because:

- he is not getting enough milk at each feed
- he has a medical problem, such as reflux, that prevents him from being able to take enough milk at each feed
- he is suffering from excessive wind or colic, which keeps him awake (but does not mean he is hungry)

If you think it is better to feed totally on demand and not attempt to establish any routine at all, you should also be aware of the following:

- A baby will wake and cry for all sorts of reasons, of which hunger is only one. If you always assume that hunger is waking him you may end up feeding a baby who is crying with another problem (such as colic), which may be made worse if you feed him.

- A baby will suck on anything that you put in his mouth, so the fact that he might suck on your breast for hours on end does not necessarily mean that he is hungry, or even that he is getting any milk.
- If your baby uses your breast as a source of comfort rather than need, he may lose his ability to settle himself.
- If you feed your baby every time he is a bit peckish rather than waiting until he is genuinely hungry, you will merely teach him to snack.
- It is hard for a mother to appreciate exactly what feeding on demand (using no guidelines) involves until she tries it. Only then will she realise that feeding two-hourly, for example, does not necessarily give her two hours free until the next feed. Feeds are timed from the point at which you start feeding (because a baby normally takes most of the milk at the beginning of the feed), rather than the point at which you finish, so if a feed lasts an hour, you will only have a gap of one hour until the next feed.
- Feeding this often can make a mother so exhausted by the demands of her baby that her milk supply may dwindle rather than increase.
- A baby that is fed three- to four-hourly will usually start sleeping through the night sooner than a baby who is fed for weeks on end at totally random times, with his mother making no attempt to space out feeds.

Feeding on a strict four-hourly schedule (I do not recommend this)

In my experience mothers tend to fall into two main categories:

1. Those who are very relaxed and easy-going and who are perfectly prepared to feed their baby as and when he needs it, without worrying too much when he feeds and when he sleeps – i.e. they are happy to take life as it comes.
2. Those who like routine and order in their lives and want to get their babies onto a strict feeding routine right from the outset.

I think the middle road is best. Too lax an attitude to feeding and sleep times will often cause babies to become very unsettled and slow to sleep through the night; too strict a routine may not suit every baby and will create a lot of stress all round.

For at least the first two or three weeks you are unlikely to establish any kind of a routine, other than trying not to feed your baby too often (i.e. preferably not more than nine times a day). But once your milk supply is well established, you can start trying to ease him into a better feeding pattern if he hasn't already got into one of his own accord.

Suggestions that might improve feeding times:

● Check whether your milk supply is good and try to increase it if it isn't (see page 87).

- Make sure you are feeding your baby for long enough at each feed and not letting him fall asleep before he has had enough milk.
- If your baby is suffering from excessive wind, colic or anything else that is making him uncomfortable, see your GP who may be able to prescribe something that will help.
- If you have a very 'sucky' baby who needs the comfort of something to suck on in between feeds, try using a dummy. But do not give a dummy to a baby who might be hungry – he needs food, not a dummy! (For more advice on dummies, see page 26.)
- Try offering water in between feeds – this may help settle him until a feed is due.

Note: You should not offer water if your milk supply is low and your baby is hungry. A hungry baby needs calories, and filling him up with water instead of milk is not the answer – not only will this affect his appetite and deprive him of essential calories but it may also prevent him feeding enough at the breast to stimulate your milk supply.

Should I wake my baby for a late-evening (10–11pm) feed?

From about six weeks onwards, many babies stop waking for the late-evening feed and gradually go longer until they need their next feed. This is the start of a baby being physically able to sleep through the night. At this point mothers face a dilemma: do they wake their baby for a 10pm feed in the hope that he will then sleep through until a civilised hour (6am, 7am or even 8am); or do they leave him to sleep and risk him waking shortly after they have gone to bed. Opinion on this is divided.

Theory one

You *should* continue to wake your baby for a late-evening feed to encourage him start sleeping through the night from a young age. Babies who are not woken for this feed tend to be slower to sleep through the night and are also more likely to get into a habit of waking earlier in the morning than babies who continue to be fed at 10pm for several months.

Theory two

You should not wake a baby for this feed as it is unfair to disrupt your baby's natural sleep pattern to suit your (rather than his) needs.

I don't think it matters either way. You should make a decision based on whatever works best for you and your baby. For example, some mothers are thrilled if their baby starts sleeping through the 10pm feed, while others would prefer to carry on doing the 10pm feed and have the longest sleep time taking place after this.

You can experiment to see what happens. If you wake your baby and he feeds well, settles back to sleep quickly and then sleeps longer as a result, it makes sense to continue waking him. But if your baby is hard to wake, feeds badly, takes ages to settle back to sleep and still wakes within a few hours it is better to leave him sleeping through the 10pm feed.

Night feeds

When breast-feeding, it is best for a mother to do all the feeds, including the ones at night. Some mothers can miss the middle-of-the-night feed without any adverse effects, but they are the exception rather than the rule. This is because:

- Most breasts need regular stimulation in the early weeks in order to establish and maintain a good supply.
- Night feeds are thought to give a greater boost to milk production than daytime feeds.
- If you miss out a night feed, your breasts may become very engorged and this can trigger off a bout of mastitis.
- If you give him formula at night (instead of expressing your own milk) you are undoing many of the health benefits of breast-feeding.

If you're desperate to catch up on some sleep, you could risk missing the occasional feed so someone else can give your baby a bottle. To do this it's best to express some extra milk during the day, both to keep your milk supply up and to provide your own milk (rather than formula) for the night feed. A better solution for tired mothers is to express a small amount of milk during the day, give your baby a quick feed from the breast when he wakes at night, then leave him to finish the feed with your expressed milk. This has the advantage of emptying most of the milk out of your breasts but you don't then have to stay up until he is fully fed and settled. Another popular solution is to express shortly before the late-evening feed – you can then have an early night and your baby is given your expressed milk when he wakes.

How to get your baby to sleep through the night
Many babies start going longer at night from about six weeks. Some do it earlier than this and others a lot later, but in general a baby will gradually reduce night feeds when he is physically ready to do so, providing he is getting plenty of milk during the day and he has no problems (such as colic or reflux) that will disrupt his sleep.

A baby who has established a good feeding pattern consisting of regular feeds and plenty of sleep in between will usually sleep better at night than a baby who is being fed totally 'on demand' without any attempt being made to establish a routine. Thus, a baby who is feeding three- to four-hourly will generally sleep through the night sooner than a baby who is 'snacking' every hour or so and cat-napping throughout the day.

Remember this: a relaxed, well-fed baby will sleep longer and better than a tense, overtired baby.

To encourage night-time sleep

- Make sure that you are offering your baby plenty of milk during the day.
- Try to space out feeds and organise your day so your baby is allowed to sleep in peace.
- Establish a routine whereby he is bathed, fed and settled quietly at a similar time each evening.
- Learn to recognise your baby's signals so you always put him down to sleep at exactly the right moment. If you put him down too early he won't be ready to drift off to sleep; if you leave it even a few minutes too late he will be overtired and will be equally unable to settle. This applies during the day as well as night.
- Put him in a quiet room to sleep in the evening.
- Distinguish between night and day by feeding your baby at night with the lights dimmed.
- Make sure that he is not getting cold at night – you may need to start using a sleeping bag during the winter months if he is coming out from under his blankets.
- Decide whether you want to wake him for a late-evening feed (see page 61) or to let him sleep through.

All of the above will work with most babies but be aware that:

- A very small or premature baby may need night feeds for a lot longer than a full-term baby.
- A baby suffering from reflux (or any other medical problem) will only sleep through when successful treatment makes him more comfortable and he can take larger feeds during the day.
- A small number of babies continue to wake at night for no obvious reason – you may just have to be patient.

I do not believe that you should try to force a baby to sleep through the night until he is six months old. After this almost all babies should be able to sleep through, so it is both reasonable and advisable to take firmer measures to achieve this if your baby is still waking – especially as it is easier to resolve bad sleeping habits in a young baby than a toddler. Tried and tested methods (such as 'controlled crying') are described in many other baby books – I do not plan to go into any more detail myself as this book is not intended to be a full child-care manual. (See 'Useful Resources', page 123, for recommended further reading.)

6 Expressing Milk and Giving Bottles

Many mothers plan to breast-feed most of the time and give bottles of expressed milk whenever they want a break (e.g. in the middle of the night). Unfortunately, this isn't always as easy as you might think. Some mothers can't do it because their breasts only produce enough milk for the baby's immediate needs and little or nothing is left at the end of a feed; others have the reverse problem of having too much milk and find that expressing over-stimulates their breasts, creating engorgement and sometimes mastitis.

Luckily, most mothers *can* combine breast-feeding with expressing and they then have the best of both worlds – their baby only receives breast milk but she does not have to do all the feeds herself.

Although it is usually best to wait until breast-feeding is well established before you start expressing, situations may arise (see page 75) that precipitate matters. For this reason, I recommend that you research the different types of breast pumps available (see page 124) and buy one in advance so that you are prepared. Breast milk can also be expressed by hand (see below), but most mothers find that this takes too long and prefer to use a pump if they are expressing on a regular basis.

The milk you express can be kept in the fridge in a sterile bottle or container for about 24 hours. You can add more expressed milk to milk that you have expressed earlier on in the day, but if you do this, the expiry time for the milk will be 24 hours from the *first* milk you expressed. Breast milk can also be frozen for about three months in special freezer bags that you can buy from chemists.

Note: Recommendations for the length of time that breast milk can safely be stored in a fridge vary from 24 hours to eight days. I prefer to err on the side of caution and advise my clients to use the milk within 24 hours. Any milk not used within 24 hours should be thrown away.

How to express by hand
This is a skill which some mothers master more easily than others, but it is relatively easy once you know how to do it. If you find it difficult, ask your midwife to show you.

- Stimulate your let-down reflex by gently stroking your breast from the top down towards your nipple.
- After about 10 strokes you can start squeezing the areola well behind your nipple (using your thumb and first finger), squeezing and releasing alternately until drops of milk appear on your nipple.

- Lean slightly forward and continue squeezing and releasing, allowing the milk to squirt or drip into a sterile container.
- Swap breasts when the milk flow slows down.
- Carry on doing this until you have expressed enough milk for your needs or until your breasts are empty.

How to express with a pump
- Sit comfortably (you do not need to lean forwards).
- Hand express to stimulate your milk flow (as described above).
- Then apply the pump, making sure your nipple is central in the funnel.
- If the funnel comes with a soft plastic insert, experiment to see whether it is more comfortable to use the pump with or without it (this will depend on the size and shape of your breast).
- Hold the funnel close enough to your breast to maintain suction, but not so close that it digs into your breast and squashes your milk ducts.
- Switch the pump on and gradually increase the suction until your milk starts flowing. Don't traumatise your nipple by having the suction too high – expressing should not hurt.
- Swap breasts whenever your milk slows down – you can keep swapping back and forth until you have enough milk and/or your breasts are empty.

Note: A breast pump allows a mother to see for herself the huge variations in milk flow. Many are surprised to see that their milk squirts out from one or more ducts on the surface of their nipple, while others are dismayed to see that their milk drips out really slowly. Both speeds are totally normal and explain why some mothers can feed their babies much more quickly than others.

What time of day should I express?
There is no set time of day that is ideal for expressing milk. Each mother needs to discover for herself at which point of the day she has the most milk (this tends to be in the morning) and to see whether it suits her to express milk at this time. It is better to express straight after, rather than before, a feed to give your breasts time to fill up again before the next feed.

Expressing myths
Mothers are given lots of contradictory advice on expressing so it can be hard to know which advice is correct. These are five of the most common misconceptions and the thinking that lies behind the different views:

1. You must not express for the first six weeks
The reasoning behind this advice seems to be that expressing before the milk supply is fully established will affect the delicate balance of

supply and demand and may stimulate the breasts to over-produce. I agree that this could happen, but only if the mother is expressing excessively and is taking far more milk out of her breasts than her baby is actually drinking. Expressing should not cause a problem if the mother is doing it in order to give the milk to her baby in a bottle – e.g. because he can't latch on, she has sore nipples, or she simply wants someone else to give a feed occasionally.

2. You must not express if your breasts are engorged

Many mothers suffer from extreme engorgement when their milk first comes in around day four, but are often advised that on no account should they express as this will make the engorgement even worse. This is bad advice. When a mother is in agony from primary engorgement and her baby is unable to empty her breasts, it is important that she *does* fully empty both breasts with a breast pump (see 'Primary engorgement', page 82).

3. Long-term expressing will reduce your milk supply

I disagree. Many mothers who cannot breast-feed their baby (because he is unable to suck on the breast for whatever reason) *are* able to express for months on end and have no problem with maintaining their supply. But it is equally true that others find that their milk supply *does* dwindle and they have to supplement with some formula milk. But the same applies to mothers who are breast-feeding – some have plenty of milk and others don't. It does not make sense to blame long-term expressing for a failing milk supply!

4. A baby will always get more milk out of a breast than a pump

Not true! Most good breast pumps are very effective at emptying a breast and will often do a far better job than a sleepy baby. I regularly express milk at the end of a feed when the baby won't suck any more on the breast but is still hungry and unsettled – the baby *will* then take this milk from a bottle.

5. If you can't express any milk, your breasts must be empty

This is generally correct. A pump normally gives a pretty good indication of your milk supply: the more milk you can express, the more you have; the less milk you express, the less you have. But if you are one of the *very* few mothers who can never express any milk (even before a feed when you know your breasts are full), using a pump to see how much milk is in your breasts is clearly not an option.

How to give top-up bottles (and express afterwards)

A top-up bottle is the best way to offer extra milk to a hungry and/or unsettled breast-fed baby, and expressing immediately after a feed allows you to see why your baby needed more milk from a bottle; is it because he is not sucking effectively, because you don't have enough milk, or is it a mixture of the two?

This is what you do:

- Breast-feed your baby for as long as he is sucking properly or for a maximum of an hour.
- Then offer him as much milk as he wants, making sure that some milk is left in the bottle – so you know he has stopped feeding because he is full rather than because you have run out of milk.
- Ideally you would offer him milk that you have expressed earlier on that day, or retrieved from the freezer. If you can't express enough milk for him (which is very likely if your supply is low), you will have to use formula.
- As soon as he has finished feeding, you need to express so you can see how much milk is left in the breast compared with the amount he has just drunk from the bottle.

Diagnosis:

- If you can't get as much out as he has just taken from the bottle, your milk supply is low and you will need to keep giving top-ups until you can improve it (see 'Not enough milk', page 87).
- If you can get plenty out, your baby is not breast-feeding effectively and you will need to continue offering top-ups until his sucking improves.

Note: You should express every time your baby has a top-up. If you don't do this your breasts will be under-stimulated and your supply will get worse. Any milk you express can be given at subsequent feeds.

Introducing a bottle

I think it is very important that all breast-fed babies get used to drinking from a bottle as well as the breast. I regularly see mothers who are distraught because their baby will not feed at all from a bottle. This can cause real problems because:

- she has to go back to work
- her milk supply is dwindling and her baby's weight gain is poor
- her baby is constantly hungry, waking at night etc., yet he refuses to take extra milk from a bottle
- she wants to attend an important event (e.g. a wedding) and can't easily take the baby with her

To stop this problem arising I *strongly* recommend that from about three weeks onwards you start substituting the occasional breast-feed with a bottle of expressed milk. This will not make your baby reject your breast but will give you peace of mind that your baby is not totally reliant on you for all his feeds. As virtually every breast-fed baby will end up having a bottle at some point, here are a few tips:

- Most bottles suit most babies.
- Experiment with different bottles if your baby is feeding badly or 'messily'.
- Only buy an expensive 'anti-colic' bottle if you *know* your baby suffers from colic or wind.
- You don't need to use specially designed 'breast-shaped' teats if you are mixing breast-feeding and bottle-feeding.
- There is little to choose nutritionally from the various brands of formula milk.
- Follow the manufacturers' instructions on making up and storing feeds.
- See page 54 for guidelines on how much milk your baby needs.

More detailed information on bottle-feeding (and bottle rejection) is contained in *What to Expect When You're Breast-feeding...and What If You Can't?* and *Top Tips for Bottle-feeding*.

7 Common Feeding Problems for Mothers

I do not recommend that this chapter should be read in great detail during the ante-natal period. Most of it is really only relevant to a mother who is actually having one of the problems described, and reading too much about potential problems is more likely to be off-putting than helpful! Instead, I suggest that you just glance at the different subjects covered so that you will know where to look if you need help after your baby is born.

Baby can't latch on
This is an extremely common problem and is usually caused by:

- a mother having large, flat or inverted nipples
- the baby being very small or premature so he physically can't open his mouth wide enough to get the nipple in his mouth
- the baby having a poor sucking reflex or tongue-tie, which makes him push your nipple out rather than suck it in
- the mother's technique is wrong!

Over the years I have had many tearful phone calls from mothers who can't latch their baby onto the breast and this is one of my favourite problems to deal with. I can usually (but not always) latch the baby on within a few seconds; one parent who didn't believe that I could do it so quickly, surreptitiously timed me to see how long it took – luckily I lived up to my reputation on that occasion! A bit less 'nose-to-nipple and skin-to-skin' and a bit more 'shaping-and-shoving' is usually all it takes. So, if your baby can't latch on, do not despair, but instead re-read the latching-on section (pages 13–17). If this doesn't help, try using nipple shields (see below) or expressing.

Using a nipple shield

If your baby can't latch on using my 'shape and shove' method, your next best option is to try using a nipple shield. The shape of the shield makes latching on easier, and the suction exerted by your baby will often pull your nipple into a better shape. If this happens, try removing the nipple shield after a few minutes to see whether he can now latch on. If he can't, you can use the nipple shield for the entire feed, providing your milk flows well enough through it for your baby to get the milk as easily. If your feeds don't last too long and your baby's weight gain is fine, you could continue using nipple shields for weeks or even months on end.

If you do try using shields, it is important to understand *how* to use them so that your baby gets enough milk and your supply isn't adversely affected. These are the main rules:

- You should not use shields before your milk comes in as your baby will be unable to get colostrum through the shields.
- Select the right size shield. A small baby will need a small shield (available from Medela) while bigger babies can use pretty much any size or make of shield. The size of the shield required is dependent on the size of your baby's mouth, *not* on the size of your nipples.
- You must check that your baby is actually getting milk when he sucks on the shields. If you are lucky enough to have a fast flow of milk you will hear your baby swallowing and you will see plenty of milk inside the shield when you take him off.
- If your milk flows slowly and there is little or no sign of milk inside the shield, you should stop using them.
- You should also stop using shields if your feeds start becoming longer and your baby is less contented and/or is not gaining enough weight.
- If your baby *is* feeding well and gaining weight, you can continue to use a shield for as long as this continues to be the case, as it clearly is not reducing your milk supply. Many mothers are able to use a shield for months.
- Nipple shields should either be sterilised or washed thoroughly and kept in a clean container.

Expressing

If nipple shields don't work, your final option is to express (see Chapter 6 'Expressing Milk and Giving Bottles').

- Try using the pump for a few minutes immediately before you feed to see whether it pulls your nipple into a better shape. If it does, stop pumping and quickly try to latch him on while your nipple is still sticking out.
- If your baby still can't latch, express all your milk and give it to him in a bottle, then try again at the next feed.
- If the problem continues, try to get one step ahead with your expressing so your hungry baby doesn't have to wait while you express his feed. Every time he fails to latch on, you should give him milk you have expressed earlier (or formula if you don't have any) and then empty your breasts with a pump ready for the next feed. The milk you express should be kept in the fridge and then warmed before it is given to him.

You can continue doing this until your baby does latch on or until you feel it is a lost cause and he is never going to manage it. At this point you need to decide whether you are willing and able to carry on expressing or whether you should call it a day and go onto bottle-feeding with formula. The decision has to be yours.

Sore nipples
This is an extremely common problem and is one of the main reasons why so many mothers stop breast-feeding. If breast-feeding is painful you should not accept it as part and parcel of breast-feeding, but instead try to resolve the problem as soon as possible.

Sore nipples are mainly caused by:

- Incorrect latching on at the breast. Many midwives cannot recognise a poor latch, so do not assume that your baby is latched on correctly just because you have been told he is!
- The excessively long feeds that can result from incorrect positioning. If your baby sucks for hours on end (especially during the first few days) but never seems satisfied, he probably isn't latched on well enough to get your milk. And bad latching causes sore nipples.
- Nipples infected with thrush or other skin problems (see page 81).
- White nipple (see page 82).
- A mother having exceptionally delicate nipples (this is fairly rare).

If you can rule out obvious problems (such as thrush), you should focus all your efforts into getting the baby to latch on better, as this is easily the main reason a mother suffers pain. When I show a mother how to latch her baby on correctly, she is usually amazed that her feeds instantly become pain-free, even though her nipples are still cracked and sore! If you cannot find anyone to improve your latching-on technique, read (and re-read!) the section in this book describing how to shape your breast to help your baby to latch on correctly (see page 16).

My DVD *Breastfeeding Without Tears* also shows this technique in great detail and is available by mail order on 01624 640000.

Tips that will also help include:

- Use a good nipple cream (e.g. Lansinoh).
- Express your milk for a few feeds and give it to your baby in a bottle. This will give your breasts a break and allow your nipples to heal.
- Try using nipple shields. If you have a good flow of milk, the shields will protect your nipples and your baby should still get your milk easily (see page 76).

Once your nipples have recovered, you may find that they have also toughened up and you can go back to full breast-feeding, even if your technique is still not perfect. But if the cracks and soreness return, improving your baby's latch is the only answer. The alternative is to continue expressing or using shields.

Thrush

It is very common for mothers and/or babies to get thrush, especially after taking antibiotics.

Signs and symptoms

- cracked and/or sore nipples that don't heal
- sore nipples that suddenly develop after a period of pain-free breast-feeding
- the nipple and areola are pink, shiny and itchy
- intense pain as the baby sucks, which feels like broken glass
- shooting pains in the breast, either during or after feeding
- white spots in the baby's mouth
- a thick, creamy white coating on his tongue, usually on the back half, which does not rub off
- nappy rash that does not heal

If you think you have thrush you should see your GP, who will be able to make a diagnosis and prescribe a suitable treatment. You can carry on breast-feeding during treatment and the thrush will usually clear up within a few days. Any milk that you have expressed (and possibly frozen) during an episode of thrush should be thrown away, as this may re-infect you and/or your baby. You should also be meticulous with hygiene and be sure to sterilise all feeding equipment.

White nipple

This is a condition that may be associated with circulatory problems. When the baby feeds, the blood drains from the nipple causing intense pain and blanching of the nipple. Poor attachment of the baby to the breast and feeding in a cold room will often be the trigger for this. In severe cases your GP might need to prescribe a drug to improve circulation.

Primary engorgement

When the milk first comes in (around day three or four) some women find that their breasts become extremely hard, painful and engorged with too much milk. This happens when the breasts fill up with milk faster than the baby empties them, either because the breasts are over-producing or because the baby is not latching on well enough to empty the breasts effectively. You can also get engorged if you miss out some feeds (e.g. at night) or if your milk comes in *very* quickly.

Prevention

- Ensure that your baby latches on correctly.
- Do not miss night feeds as day four approaches.
- If your baby has been unable to latch on and is being fed with formula milk, start expressing your milk as soon as it begins to come in.

Treatment

- Express a bit of milk (by hand or with a pump) to soften the area behind your nipple and make it easier for your baby to latch on.
- Try using a nipple shield (if your baby can't latch on).
- If your baby can't extract the milk (either through a nipple shield or directly from the breast) your breasts will feel just as hard and uncomfortable at the end of the feed as they did at the start. Your baby will also appear hungry and unsettled even though he may have spent a long time sucking on the breast. If this happens, you should express your milk with a pump and offer it to your baby in a bottle – you will need to keep doing this until he manages to empty the breast himself.
- If your baby *is* getting all the milk he needs but your breasts are still rock hard and solid at the end of the feed it is essential to express to avoid getting mastitis. If you empty your breasts fully once or twice (i.e. until they are soft and comfortable) the problem is usually resolved instantly.
- But if your breasts continue to fill up as fast as you empty them, you should *not* keep expressing as this will stimulate your supply and make the engorgement worse. Instead, leave your breasts to regulate themselves (this normally takes a few days) and take antibiotics if you develop mastitis.
- Taking a mild painkiller such as paracetamol and putting cold

cabbage leaves or special gel pads (available from chemists) into your bra will help reduce the pain and inflammation.
- A good supporting bra with wide shoulder straps is essential.

Many mothers are told that on no account must they express as this will only make the engorgement worse. This is simply not true! Expressing to relieve extreme engorgement does not stimulate the milk supply. But if breasts are left to become severely engorged, lactation may be suppressed, resulting in neither the baby nor a breast pump being able to get any milk out of the breasts. The mother may then find it hard to build up her milk supply once the engorgement subsides.

Mastitis

This commonly occurs as a result of severe engorgement, poor latching, sore nipples or blocked milk ducts. A mild bout of mastitis will usually cause few problems, but severe mastitis can make a mother feel very ill, reduce her milk supply and, if left untreated, may develop into an abscess.

Signs and symptoms of mastitis
- blocked milk ducts
- part of the breast becomes hard, lumpy and painful, and doesn't soften up after feeding

- a red patch or red streaks on the breast, which may also feel hot and painful
- aching, flu-like symptoms and a high temperature

Treatment
- Use a breast pump to try and empty the breast and get rid of the lumps. If you succeed and your symptoms subside, you need do nothing further.
- If your symptoms do not improve within 12–24 hours you should see your GP as soon as possible as you will need antibiotics. The sooner you start taking them, the sooner the infection will clear up. If you avoid taking antibiotics you may develop an abscess and you will need to go to hospital to have it incised and drained.
- You can (and should) carry on breast-feeding. Don't worry if your baby develops diarrhoea as it will not harm him (unless it is very severe) and will stop as soon as you finish taking the antibiotics.
- If your baby can't or won't suck on the affected breast, use a pump at every feed to try and empty the breast and restore a good milk flow.
- It should take about 24 hours for you to start feeling better, but if there is little or no improvement after two to three days, you should see your GP again as you may need a different type of antibiotic.
- If your milk supply is badly affected you may need to give formula milk as a top-up until your supply improves. (Unfortunately for some women, the milk supply never fully recovers.)

Too much milk

If your breasts make far more milk than your baby needs, you will feel over-full and uncomfortable for several days until production slows down. For a very small number of mothers it may take several weeks for this to happen.

The following tips will help:

- Wear a good supporting bra.
- Express a *small* amount of milk in between feeds if you are excessively uncomfortable.
- Try not to express more milk than is absolutely necessary for your comfort, because expressing too often will stimulate your breasts to produce even more milk.
- If expressing small amounts doesn't help, you could try emptying the breasts completely after one or two feeds, using a breast pump. If this doesn't solve the problem (i.e. your breasts still fill up more quickly than your baby can empty them) you should not keep doing this.
- Use breast shells if your breasts are leaking a lot. These will be more effective than breast-pads and you can keep any milk that you collect.

Milk flow is too fast

Some mothers have such a fast milk flow that the baby simply can't cope and feeding becomes very traumatic. Your milk flow is too fast for your baby if:

- you can hear him gulping and choking as he feeds
- he keeps pulling off your breast and crying
- your milk continues to drip or spurt out of your breast, even when he is not sucking
- he starts refusing to latch onto your breast, even though he is clearly hungry

If this happens, try using a nipple shield. This will help by slowing and containing the flow, so your baby only gets milk when he chooses to suck. As your baby gets older he may find it easier to cope, so it's worth trying to feed him without a nipple shield every now and then to see whether he can manage without it.

Not enough milk

A poor milk supply is another of the main reasons that mothers give up breast-feeding. I regularly visit mothers who have so much milk that they could feed several babies and then I see others who have *never* had enough milk – no hint of engorgement and a hungry baby who is feeding endlessly and not gaining weight.

I firmly believe that having too much or too little milk is more a question of luck than management, and I also believe that while some women *can* improve their supply by following standard advice (resting, eating and drinking plenty, and feeding more frequently), others can't.

Your milk supply is probably low if:

- your baby is feeding endlessly and cries every time you put him down to sleep
- his weight gain is poor
- he will only settle if you give him a top-up
- you can't express any milk from your breasts after he has needed a top-up
- you substitute an entire breast-feed with a bottle-feed and then can't express as much milk out of both breasts as he has just taken from the bottle

Tips to improve your supply:

- Make sure you are eating and drinking plenty, and also that you are getting enough rest. If possible, retire to bed for a day or two, taking your baby with you. This way, you can concentrate solely on feeding him and keep your energy for making milk.

- Give your breasts the message that your baby needs more milk by feeding longer and more frequently, but take him off the breast when he is no longer sucking properly (see page 93).
- Only offer top-up bottles if you simply cannot settle your baby without one.
- Use a breast pump at the end of every feed to express any milk that might be left and to stimulate milk production – any milk you express can be given as a top-up at a subsequent feed.

It usually takes several days for things to improve and for your baby to cut down on the amount of milk that he needs as a top-up. But if you see no improvement at all after a week or so, you may have to accept that your breasts are not responding to treatment and that there is little point in continuing to try to achieve the impossible. You can still carry on breast-feeding but you should stop expressing and top-up with formula milk.

Note: There are numerous homeopathic and over-the-counter remedies that claim to boost milk production and are certainly worth trying if all else fails. Some of my clients swear by them, while others notice little or no improvement. You can try drinking four to five cups of fennel tea a day and/or take three fenugreek tablets three times a day – these remedies can be found in good health food shops and some pharmacies. However, it is best to consult a homeopath if you wish to try a homeopathic preparation as he will be able to advise you as to which remedy is best suited to you.

As a last resort, you could ask your doctor if he will prescribe Domperidone. This is a drug normally prescribed for dyspepsia, reflux oesophagitis and vomiting, but which has also been found to increase milk production in breast-feeding mothers. Domperidone is not licensed for this use (increasing milk supply), so your GP may be reluctant to prescribe it without first researching the relevant information. Some women taking Domperidone will notice an increase in milk supply within 24 hours, while others find it takes several days or even two to three weeks before a full benefit is noticed.

Please don't feel a failure if you cannot increase your milk supply. Common sense dictates that, 'if neither your baby nor a breast pump can get enough milk out of *your* breasts to give *your* baby all the milk he needs', your only option is to supplement with formula. This does *not* make you a bad mother.

Growth spurts

It is normal for a baby to have an occasional growth spurt and suddenly need a lot more milk. Growth spurts usually occur at approximately three weeks, six weeks, three months and six months. If this happens, you will need to increase your food and fluid intake, feed him more frequently and rest more until your milk supply increases to meet the new demands. This will probably take 24 to 48 hours.

Baby 'fussing' at the breast

Breast-feeding should be a peaceful and happy experience. When a mother settles down to feed her baby she expects him to latch on easily and then feed calmly until he is full. Unfortunately, it's not unusual for a baby to become very agitated at the breast – and the more he cries and fusses, the more stressful feed times can become.

Common scenarios

- It is always hard to latch your baby on. He starts crying as soon as you lie him near your breast and his head bobs back and forth while he frantically tries to latch onto the nipple. He can't manage it and the more you push him towards the breast, the more he cries and pulls away. Everyone gets fraught! This often happens if you bring your baby towards the breast at the wrong angle and/or you don't help him by shaping your nipple. This makes it hard for him to latch on and it is very frustrating for him. The hungrier he is, the more upset he will get (see 'Baby can't latch on', page 75).
- Your baby latches on easily, but almost immediately starts crying and pulling away. This tends to happen when your milk flows too fast for your baby to cope (see page 87).
- Your baby feeds well but then starts crying and pulling off the breast towards the end of the feed, even though you think he is

still hungry. Your milk may be flowing too slowly or your breast may be empty (see page 87).

- Your baby starts feeding well but then cries and pulls off the breast frequently throughout the feed and appears to be in pain. Your baby may be suffering from wind (see page 22), colic (see page 105) or reflux (see page 109).

- Feeding has gone well for weeks or even months and then, for no apparent reason, your baby starts crying and fussing at the breast. Typically, he will latch on well but at some point will cry and arch his back and pull away from your breast, often dragging your nipple in his mouth. Sometimes he will latch on again almost immediately and at other times you have to spend ages calming him down before he will go back to the breast. This behaviour may only last for a few feeds and then miraculously stop, or it may go on for days until you reach the point where you contemplate giving up breast-feeding. Unfortunately, I don't know why babies do this. It may be that the mother has eaten something (such as garlic) that is making her breast milk taste unpleasant. It could also be that the mother is suffering from stress or has started taking a lot of exercise, both of which (according to recent research) can affect the taste of the milk. Apart from suggesting that you examine your lifestyle and diet, making any necessary changes, there is little that I can advise other than to 'muddle' through and hope that this behaviour doesn't persist for too long.

Note: If your baby appears unwell and/or is not gaining weight, consult your GP.

Is your diet affecting your baby?
When breast-feeding, a mother should be able to eat pretty much whatever she wants, as very few foods will affect her baby via the breast milk. But if you notice that your baby regularly becomes unsettled, windy or colicky every time you eat a certain food, it is best to cut it out of your diet for as long as you are breast-feeding. If your baby is only being affected by one or two foods which commonly affect babies (e.g. citrus fruits, curry or garlic), there is no need to consult a doctor. But if your baby is showing signs of milk allergy or lactose intolerance (see pages 114 and 115) you should see your GP.

Baby can't or won't suck efficiently
Most babies are born with a strong sucking reflex, but a small number can't or won't suck on the breast. Some of these babies will even be slow to feed from a bottle.

With skilled help, it normally only takes a few feeds for the baby to improve his technique, but occasionally it takes days or even weeks before breast-feeding is fully established.

The first step is to diagnose the problem and then see whether anything can be done about it. Some babies can't latch on at all, while others either fall asleep after a few sucks or suck in such a feeble way that they get little or no milk.

This can be caused by any of the following:

- Your baby is latched on badly and is therefore not getting the milk easily.
- Your baby is dehydrated and has no energy to suck.
- He is jaundiced and is too sleepy to feed.
- He is a naturally sleepy baby and needs regular stimulation to keep him feeding.
- Your nipple is so big and hard (like a marble) that he genuinely can't get enough of it into his small mouth.
- He was born prematurely and needs time to develop a stronger sucking reflex.
- He has a minor defect (such as tongue-tie) which prevents him sucking efficiently.
- He suffered intracranial trauma at birth (minor damage to his head) which is affecting his sucking reflex. A cranial osteopath may be able to resolve this problem (see page 117).
- He has an infection that needs diagnosing and treating.
- You have little or no milk and your baby is not prepared to suck on an empty breast.

By referring to the relevant sections in this book you should find that you can resolve most of the above issues. However, I do occasionally come across a healthy full-term baby who simply will not suck on the breast even though he has no problems latching on and the mother has plenty of milk. It is extremely frustrating when this happens but, as I say to the mother, 'You can take a horse to water, but you can't make him drink!' With these babies, I will suggest the mother expresses her milk and gives it in a bottle until such time as his sucking gets better or the mother feels she can't carry on expressing.

The ill mother
It is normally safe to continue breast-feeding if you are suffering from a common illness such as a cold or flu, but if you develop a more unusual illness (e.g. food poisoning) you should consult a doctor. If he advises you to stop breast-feeding for a few days, you will need to express at least four-hourly (and throw the milk away) in order to keep your milk supply going until you can start again. In the meantime, your baby can be fed with formula milk. Mothers who are HIV- or Hepatitis-positive are advised not to breast-feed at all.

8 Common Feeding Problems for Babies

As with the previous chapter, I feel it would be counter-productive to read the whole of this one during the ante-natal period, as it also concentrates on problems, and, with a bit of luck, you will not have to read it at all! None the less, it is still worth flicking through the headings so that you know which problems are covered, in case you experience any of them and find that you do need help.

Jaundice
It is very common and normal for a baby to become jaundiced within the first few days and in most cases this clears up of its own accord within two weeks without the need for any treatment. Jaundice occurs when there is more bilirubin in the blood than the liver can cope with, creating a build-up of bilirubin in the body, which turns the baby's skin and eyes yellow.

A baby is more likely to become severely jaundiced and need treatment if:

- he is very small or premature
- he suffered trauma and bruising during delivery (e.g. after a forceps or ventouse extraction)
- he becomes dehydrated because he is not breast-feeding well

You do not need to worry if your baby is only mildly jaundiced and is feeding well, but you should contact your community midwife (or even take your baby back to hospital) if:

- the jaundice is increasing (i.e. your baby is becoming a darker yellow and it is spreading from his face and eyes down to the rest of his body)
- he is very sleepy, difficult to rouse, and reluctant to feed
- he is showing signs of dehydration (see page 48)

Jaundice should always be taken seriously because very high levels of bilirubin can (very rarely) cause permanent brain damage.

If in doubt, you should take your baby to hospital for a blood test as this is the only completely accurate way of finding out whether his jaundice needs treating. If his bilirubin levels are too high, he will need to be admitted to hospital for a day or two for phototherapy.

If your baby is only mildly jaundiced, you should make sure that he is fed regularly (at least three- to four-hourly) until the jaundice fades.

Note: If he is too sleepy to feed efficiently from the breast, you may need to express your milk and bottle-feed him for a few feeds.

Breast milk jaundice
A very small number of babies will develop breast milk jaundice, thought to be caused by the mother having an enzyme in her milk that temporarily stops the bilirubin being expelled effectively. This jaundice is usually mild and does no harm and the bilirubin levels will gradually return to normal over a period of three to 10 weeks. If there is any cause for concern, blood tests can be done to exclude liver or thyroid problems, but in most cases the mother can carry on breast-feeding until the condition resolves itself.

Note: If you stop breast-feeding for a couple of days breast milk jaundice will usually disappear very quickly, but it is not normally necessary to do this.

The sleepy baby
Having a sleepy, contented baby is a real bonus to tired mothers. But if your baby is too sleepy to feed properly and is not gaining weight, re-read the above section on jaundice, as well as the sections on dehydration (page 48) and poor weight gain (page 103) to see what to do.

Note: If your baby remains abnormally sleepy, you should consult a doctor – he may have an infection (e.g. of the urinary tract) that requires treatment.

The unsettled baby
Coping with a crying, unsettled baby, who is constantly demanding attention, is tiring, stressful and extremely demoralising. Worse still, most parents don't know *why* their baby is crying, nor do they know what to do about it.

If I could get only one message across to one and all it is this: **the main reason a baby cries is because he is hungry.** Unfortunately, many parents (and midwives) assume that every breast-fed baby is getting plenty of milk whenever he feeds, so the longer he feeds, the more milk he is getting. This is not true! (See 'How will I know when my baby has had enough milk?' page 21.)

If your baby is only unsettled for a small part of the occasional day, you may simply have a baby who requires a bit more attention at these times. But if your baby is constantly feeding, crying every time you put him down and will only stop if you cuddle him or take him into bed with you – don't struggle on. Instead, re-read Chapter 2 on how to feed and settle your baby. You should also refer to the sections on colic, reflux and milk allergy, (pages 105, 109 and 114), consulting a doctor where necessary.

You should also:

- Exclude hunger by offering your baby extra milk as a top-up bottle. If he takes some milk and then falls sound asleep, your problem is solved. If he rejects the bottle, at least you have established that he is not hungry and there is no point continuing to put him to the breast.
- Make sure you are winding him properly.
- Swaddle him, offer him a dummy and rock him to sleep.
- Leave him for a few minutes to see whether he needs to cry himself to sleep (see page 25).
- Take him for a walk in his pram.
- Settle your baby to sleep on your lap (see below).

How to settle your baby on your lap

If your baby has become really fraught and overtired, settling him to sleep on your lap is a good solution. This three-step method works far better than endlessly pacing the room, swapping your baby from shoulder to shoulder, and continually putting him down as soon as he dozes off, only to find he is awake again within minutes. The real key to the success of the 'lap' method is that it tends to send your baby into a deeper and more permanent sleep than other methods and it can be done whenever you can't, or don't want to, go out with the pram. It works extremely well with babies up to the age of about three months. Babies older than this will usually settle best when taken for a long walk in a pram.

Step one

Sit comfortably with someone or something (e.g. the television!) to keep you company so that you don't try to rush things. Place a pillow on your lap and lie your baby on his tummy on the pillow, turning his head gently to one side so that you can, if necessary, put a dummy in his mouth (see below). You should then start patting your baby on his back just above the nappy level, firmly and rhythmically, at a rate of approximately one pat per second. Most babies find this very soothing and comforting and will usually fall asleep quite quickly. Don't be discouraged if he cries a lot for the first few minutes because, if you persist with the rhythmic patting, you will find that his crying will diminish and he'll start to fall asleep.

Once your baby is asleep, you can stop patting him but you should leave him lying on your lap for a few minutes longer to check that he has gone into a sound sleep and has not just dozed off. If he starts stirring and waking, pat him again (but do not pick him up) until he goes back to sleep. If he stays asleep for approximately five minutes after you have stopped patting him, you can pick him up gently and put him into his crib.

Hopefully he will remain asleep, but if he does wake up, you will need to put him back on your lap and start the process all over again.

Step two

If your baby wakes every time you move him to his crib, you may need to leave him sleeping on the pillow until his next feed is due. Gently lift the pillow from your lap and put it (and your baby) on a surface where he will be safe (e.g. on a sofa, surrounded by cushions) and not at risk of rolling off.

Step three

If your baby is so tense and overtired that he wakes every time you move the pillow, you will have to spend an hour or more sitting with him asleep on your lap. Although this is very restricting for you, it is a great deal more relaxing than the alternative of pacing around with your baby over your shoulder. You may also find that you only need to do this after one or two feeds to break the cycle of 'overtiredness' and from then on your baby will be able to settle himself.

It is safe to leave your baby to sleep on his tummy during the day, provided you are around to keep an eye on him. Do not leave him unattended.

Poor weight gain

If your baby is not gaining enough weight, he is not getting enough milk – it's as simple as that!

This may be for any of the following reasons:

- He is not feeding long enough or frequently enough. Wake him at least four-hourly (or even three-hourly) for feeds and try to keep him feeding longer.
- He is not sucking efficiently.
- Your milk supply is low, so he can't get enough milk regardless of how long or how frequently he feeds.
- He has a medical problem (e.g. reflux) that prevents him from taking the milk he wants and needs.
- His weight is being measured against charts that are appropriate for formula-fed (rather than breast-fed) babies.

As mentioned in previous chapters, the quickest and easiest way to identify the problem is to offer him a top-up from a bottle at the end of each feed:

- If he takes extra milk and his weight gain quickly improves, this shows that he was not getting enough milk.
- If you can't express as much milk as he has just taken it means your supply is low. If you *can* express the same amount, it shows he is not sucking efficiently.
- If he refuses extra milk and is crying and unsettled, he may be suffering from reflux (or other problems) and you should consult a doctor.

If his poor weight gain is due to a lack of milk, you should continue to offer top-ups and try to improve your milk supply (see page 88).

Colic
Colic is the term used to describe the pain a baby suffers when he gets griping spasms in his small intestine, which can happen before, during and after feeds. Colic affects both breast- and formula-fed babies and there is no known cause or treatment. It usually starts round about the third week and lasts for three to four months before clearing up of its own accord. Coping with a colicky baby is extremely stressful for the whole family (as well as your baby) and for this reason it is vital to get a proper diagnosis to be sure that colic really is the cause of your baby's distress.

I have seen hundreds of parents who have consulted me, claiming their baby has terrible colic when this has proved not to be so – in almost every case the problem has been either hunger or reflux. **I cannot stress enough the importance of ruling out hunger or reflux before resigning yourself (and your baby) to several months of misery.**

Signs and symptoms of colic

- The baby usually feeds well from the breast and/or bottle (often falling asleep at the end of the feed) but then wakes shortly after you put him down.
- He appears to have been woken by a sudden griping pain.
- As he cries, he may either draw his legs up to his stomach or hold them out so his whole body goes rigid.
- His abdomen may feel tense and swollen.
- Winding may help a bit but does not solve the problem (because the pain of colic is caused by a combination of wind and bowel spasms).
- Putting him back to the breast stops him crying for a bit (he is comforted by the sucking) but it does not send him to sleep.
- He refuses top-up bottles (because he is not hungry).
- Nothing stops him crying, other than holding him, rocking him or walking him in a pram.
- The baby starts crying again almost as soon as you stop walking him in the pram.

Although you cannot cure colic, there are ways of making it more bearable for both you and your baby:

- Omit any foods from your diet that may be upsetting him.
- Try the various over-the-counter remedies that are available from chemists (e.g. gripe water, Infacol or Colief).

- Ask your doctor if he can prescribe an anti-spasmodic medicine.
- Experiment with different bottles and teats. The Doctor Brown bottle may help.
- Give your baby a dummy to suck on in between feeds.
- Try not to feed him within three hours of the start of the previous feed. If you keep putting milk into his tummy, his colic is likely to become worse.
- Check that his clothing is not too tight – trousers with an elastic waistband will be more uncomfortable than a babygro, dungarees etc.
- Carry him around in a sling or take him for long walks in his pram.
- Consult a homeopath and/or a cranial osteopath.

Remember: if all else fails, your baby *will* grow out of colic eventually – usually at around three to four months.

Evening colic / evening fretting

Many babies become unsettled in the evening. Colic is sometimes to blame, but it is more likely that the baby is hungry or overtired. It is fairly common for a mother's milk supply to diminish towards the end of the day, with the result that her baby can't always get as much milk in the evening as he does the rest of the day. If this happens, you may need to give him a top-up bottle and use a breast pump to try to boost milk production.

Note: Many mothers find that giving a bottle at this time of the day (and not expressing) does not interfere with milk production during the rest of the 24 hours, but does give the baby the extra milk he needs.

Constipation

The stools of a breast-fed baby are usually more liquid and less bulky than those of a bottle-fed baby. It is perfectly normal for a baby to empty his bowels several times a day and it is also fine for him to go three or four days without doing a dirty nappy; so long as your baby is comfortable and his stools are soft, he is not constipated. You only need to worry about constipation if your baby goes for several days without passing a motion and then strains to produce stools that are hard and pellet-shaped.

Treatment

- Offer him cool, boiled water from a bottle in between feeds.
- If this doesn't help, try adding a teaspoon of brown sugar to the water.
- The most effective remedy is an ounce or two of diluted prune juice or freshly squeezed orange juice.

If his constipation is only temporary and is easily resolved with these home remedies, there is nothing further that needs to be done, but if it persists you should consult a doctor.

Anal stenosis
A very small number of babies have a tight anal sphincter muscle (anal stenosis) which makes it harder for them to pass motions, even though the stools are soft. If your baby is uncomfortable and colicky and keeps visibly straining to do a dirty nappy, but then produces soft stools, he may have anal stenosis. Not all GPs are familiar with this condition so he may need to refer you to a paediatrician who will know what to do. Treatment is very simple (it involves gently dilating the sphincter muscle) but it is not something that you should attempt to do yourself.

Tongue-tie
A baby is described as being 'tongue-tied' when the membrane that attaches the tongue to the floor of the mouth is too short and tight, and extends too far towards the tip of the tongue. This prevents the tongue from moving freely, which may make it difficult for your baby to breast-feed correctly. If this happens, you should discuss it with your doctor who may suggest that you get the tongue-tie clipped. This is painless and simple to do.

Gastro-oesophageal reflux
This is a fairly common condition that affects many babies but

frequently goes undiagnosed. Reflux happens when a baby has a weak sphincter muscle at the top of his stomach – this weakness can cause milk and acidic gastric juices to go back up into his oesophagus rather than staying in his stomach. This gives the baby the equivalent of acid heartburn every time he feeds – and the bigger the feed, the more pain he will suffer.

Many people (including doctors) will only consider reflux as a possibility if the baby is bringing up some or most of his feeds, but in reality, many babies can have severe reflux without ever being seen to vomit up milk. Instead, the milk just goes up and down in the oesophagus, with the stomach acid 'burning' and damaging the delicate tissue which lines the oesophagus – this 'silent' reflux is usually far more painful than visible reflux.

You should consider reflux if your baby is showing any of the following signs:

- He starts each feed sucking eagerly and well, but then becomes distressed as the feed progresses.
- Typically he will start crying, throwing his head back and arching his back. His whole body may become rigid and it will take several minutes to calm him down.
- He may then refuse to continue feeding, even though he has only taken a small amount of milk.
- He cries after every feed (and usually throughout the feed).

- He will become very distressed if you lay him flat on his back, and he will only stop crying when you hold him upright.
- He brings up more milk after each feed than you would expect with a normal posset.
- He consistently takes small feeds, which last him less than three hours.
- His weight gain is poor but he won't drink more milk.

When a baby is being breast-fed, it can be quite hard to diagnose reflux, as many of the above signs and symptoms can occur as a result of breast-feeding problems as well as the effects of reflux. So, in order to help you make a diagnosis, I suggest that you express your milk and give a few feeds by bottle rather than breast – this way you can see exactly what is happening.

Although some babies suffer from reflux at a very early age (even within the first week) and are difficult to feed from the outset, the majority of babies gradually become worse at feeding, with the symptoms becoming more obvious from about six weeks onwards. At this point, diagnosis becomes easier. The most obvious effect of reflux is that a baby will regularly (but not always) refuse to drink as much milk as he should be taking for his age and size. The average six-week-old baby needs a minimum of 120 ml (4 oz) per feed but more likely 150–180 ml (5–6 oz) depending on his weight. A reflux baby, on the other hand, will usually happily drink 60–90 ml (2–3 oz) and then start crying, arching his back and refusing to finish the bottle. As a baby gets older and needs larger amounts of milk, the discrepancy between the amount of milk a reflux baby will take and what he should be taking, therefore, becomes much more obvious.

If you think your baby has reflux, you should consult your GP to have the diagnosis confirmed. In obvious cases of reflux, your GP will usually prescribe Infant Gaviscon and, if you are bottle-feeding, he may also recommend you change to a special anti-reflux formula milk. If your baby improves dramatically on Gaviscon, no further treatment or tests should be necessary and he can remain on it until such time as your GP considers that it is no longer needed.

If your baby does not respond to Gaviscon or there is doubt about the diagnosis, your GP may arrange for him to go into hospital for tests – these are fairly simple and should not be too distressing for you or your baby. Depending on the results, your baby may then be prescribed an antacid such as Ranitidine or an inhibitor such as Losec, which can stop acid production altogether. Unfortunately, reflux is not always cured overnight and I'm afraid that it occasionally involves many weeks of misery (for both of you) before the right mix of drugs is found and the symptoms abate. If this does happen, try to comfort yourself with the knowledge that every baby will eventually grow out of reflux, with or without treatment.

Babies with reflux need to be kept upright as much as possible, to help keep the milk down in the stomach, so it will help if you:

- feed your baby in an upright position
- keep him sitting upright for at least half an hour after feeds
- tilt his cot by propping it up at the head end

Note: If your baby does not respond well to treatment for reflux and continues to be unable to take in enough milk for his needs, it might be a good idea to start him on solids earlier than usual (i.e. well before six months). You could discuss this with your GP or paediatrician.

Laryngomalacia

If your baby has abnormally noisy breathing, especially when feeding, he may be suffering from laryngomalacia. This is a condition where the larynx and/or the surrounding areas are under-developed and floppy.

Signs and symptoms

- The baby makes a high-pitched crowing or rattling sound on inspiration, which is usually more noticeable when he is crying, feeding or lying on his back.
- He may have difficulty in feeding and/or breathing.

Most babies grow out of this condition without needing any treatment, but you should consult a doctor if your baby is struggling to feed and is not gaining weight.

Note: Many babies with laryngomalacia also suffer from reflux.

Milk allergy / food intolerance

There is no known cause of milk allergy but it often runs in families. Milk allergy or intolerance more commonly occurs when a baby is fed formula milk, but some babies are so sensitive that they also react to a mother's diet via her breast milk.

When a baby is allergic to milk (or any food you are eating), his immune system over-reacts by producing antibodies, which cause any of the symptoms described below. These symptoms then become more immediate and more severe the longer he is exposed to milk.

Milk/food intolerance occurs when the baby finds it hard to digest milk or certain foods – it does not involve the immune system, so the symptoms are less immediate and less severe.

Signs and symptoms

- Your baby is colicky, crying and unsettled.
- He has abdominal pain and bloating.
- He suffers diarrhoea or constipation.
- He develops skin rashes or eczema.
- He has swelling around the lips or a runny nose.
- He is difficult to feed and settle, and may vomit up his feeds.

If your baby is showing any of the above signs and symptoms, you should consult a doctor to get a proper medical diagnosis. If the diagnosis is confirmed, your doctor may recommend that you exclude all dairy products from your diet and he will prescribe a specialist formula milk if you are giving any formula top-up feeds.

Most babies will eventually grow out of a milk allergy.

Lactose intolerance

Lactose is a sugar present in both breast and formula milk. It needs to be broken down by an enzyme in the bowel called lactase to allow the milk to be absorbed easily. But if a baby has little or no lactase (this can often result from a bout of gastro-enteritis) the milk is hard to digest and he may suffer from excessive wind, abdominal distension and pain, diarrhoea, frothy stools and vomiting.

If your baby is diagnosed with lactose intolerance he will need to switch to a specialist formula milk, which you may be able to get on prescription from your doctor.

Baby in neonatal intensive care unit

If your baby is initially unable to breast-feed (and has to be fed by naso-gastric tube or intravenous infusion) don't worry that this will have any long-term effect on breast-feeding. Providing you can maintain your milk supply, virtually all babies will happily revert to the breast once they are well enough to do so.

During the first few days the midwives will show you how to hand-express your colostrum and you can start using a breast pump as soon as your milk comes in – you will then need to express very regularly (at least four-hourly) in order to maintain your supply.

Most units are reluctant to give a bottle to a baby whose mother is planning to breast-feed for fear of creating 'nipple/teat confusion' (see page 51). As a result, when a baby is ready to start breast-feeding, he is usually put straight onto the breast without first checking his sucking reflex. This is fine if your baby *is* able to feed well from the breast, but not so sensible if he can't. So, if your baby is very premature and/or weak, I advise the following:

- Before trying him on the breast, you should first check to see how well he is able to suck on a bottle.
- If he feeds well from the bottle, he can start breast-feeding.
- If he shows that he *can't* suck strongly enough to take a full feed from the bottle, he certainly won't be able to get enough milk from the breast (because breast-feeding is usually harder than bottle-feeding). If this happens, you should not tire him out trying to get him on the breast.
- As soon as he shows he *can* feed well from the bottle, you can try him on the breast.
- You should then only keep him on the breast for as long as he is sucking properly (see page 20) and then offer him a top-up bottle.
- If he doesn't want any milk from the bottle, you can rest assured that he has breast-fed well.

- If he does drink some milk, you should keep offering him top-ups until he no longer needs them. You will also need to express every time your baby takes a top-up in order to maintain a good milk supply.

If you follow the above advice, most hospitals will be happy to discharge you home as soon as your baby is able to take all his feeds from breast and/or bottle. You can then gradually establish full breast-feeding as your baby gets older and stronger.

Cranial osteopathy

Osteopathy can be very successful in treating tense, irritable and unsettled babies, colic, feeding difficulties on breast or bottle, and sleeping problems. Although cranial osteopathy is very gentle and non-invasive, it is best to consult your GP and/or a breast-feeding specialist before seeing an osteopath, to rule out normal reasons for your baby's symptoms. Many babies will improve simply by changing the way you feed or handle them. It is also important to exclude medical conditions (such as reflux) before going down the road of alternative treatments for your baby.

9 How to Stop Breast-feeding

The current government recommendation is that a baby should be *exclusively* breast-fed for six months – and by this they mean no formula and no solid food during this time. In practice, very few mothers (probably less than 5 per cent) achieve this, so it is important to realise that any breast-feeding is better than none. Even if you only manage to breast-feed your baby for a week or so, you will still have given him a better start in life than a baby who has received no breast milk at all.

When the time comes to stop breast-feeding, there are several different ways to go about making the change to bottle-feeding, so you need to decide which method will work best for you. You should allow plenty of time to stop breast-feeding if you have a really good milk supply but maybe only a few days if your supply is very low and you have been giving top-ups. Allow at least three weeks for weaning if:

- you have a firm deadline for stopping breast-feeding (e.g. returning to work)
- your baby has never been given a bottle and might refuse to take one

- your milk supply is very plentiful and you become engorged whenever you miss a feed
- you are prone to mastitis
- you are planning to go on holiday without your baby – so your holiday isn't spoiled by engorged and leaking breasts!

There are three main methods of stopping breast-feeding:

1. You can miss one feed completely and substitute it with a bottle-feed. Once your breasts have adjusted to missing out this feed, you can drop another, alternating breast-feeds with bottle-feeds, rather than dropping two breast-feeds in a row. It doesn't matter which feed you drop first, but it is sensible either to drop the feed when your milk supply is at its lowest, or one that it suits you to miss (e.g. the mid-morning feed).

2. You can shorten each feed (and top-up with formula) so that your breasts are never fully emptied. The less milk your baby takes from the breast at each feed, the more quickly your breasts will reduce production.

3. You can give up breast-feeding overnight simply by stopping feeding altogether and going straight on to full-time bottle-feeding. I would not normally recommend doing this because,

although it gets it all over very quickly, there is a price to pay. Your breasts will almost certainly become engorged and painful and will remain this way for several days until they respond by halting any further milk production. It will then take a further two or three days for the milk to be re-absorbed. During this time you will feel extremely uncomfortable and you also run the risk of getting mastitis. This is not a good way to stop breast-feeding and should only be done if you don't have time to wind down more gradually.

I generally favour the first method, but for a mother who produces so much milk that she gets mastitis every time she misses a feed, stopping overnight (and taking antibiotics if she does develop mastitis) may be the only solution.

Breast-feeding and the working mother
Some mothers find it easy to continue breast-feeding when they return to work, while others can't manage it at all.

You might find any of the following issues applies to you:

- Your breasts provide plenty of milk for the first and last feed of the day and remain comfortable during the day when you are not feeding.

- Your breasts become so engorged during the day that you have to take a breast pump to work so that you can express to relieve the discomfort – this milk can then be given to your baby the following day.
- You *need* to express milk regularly throughout the day (i.e. you have no choice) in order to keep your breasts sufficiently stimulated to provide enough milk for the morning and evening feeds.
- Combining work with breast-feeding becomes too tiring and your milk supply reduces to the extent that you can no longer supply your baby with enough breast milk.

As it is impossible to predict what will happen, it really is a question of trial and error. If you are one of the unlucky ones who *does* run out of milk, you should not feel you have failed but accept that this is one of the downsides of going back to work. Your baby will be perfectly happy on formula and he will be just as happy to see you when you get home!

Useful Resources

Books

New Toddler Taming by Dr Christopher Green
This is a brilliant book. It is easy to read and contains fantastic advice on all aspects of baby and childcare. It also has an excellent section on sleep problems.

The New Contented Little Baby Book by Gina Ford
For those who would like to follow a more routine-based, step-by-step guide to caring for their baby, Gina Ford has proved invaluable to many mothers.

A Perfect Start by Christine and Peter Hill
For sound practical advice that will both help and reassure anxious new parents I thoroughly recommend this book.

DVDs
My DVD, *Breastfeeding Without Tears,* is available by mail order (Tel: 01624 640 000). On this two-hour DVD you will see me teaching an ante-natal class, and also showing mothers how to latch their baby onto the breast, as well as how to wind, swaddle etc.

Other information
Medela UK (Tel: 0161 776 0400)
Sells a huge range of breast-feeding products through mail order. I particularly recommend their breast pumps and nipple shields. They also have breast pumps for hire.

Ameda Lactaline (Tel: 01823 336 362)
I recommend their double breast pump for purchase or hire.

Babylist, 50 Sulivan Road, London SW6 3DX (Tel: 020 7371 5145)
Gives independent, unbiased advice to help you choose baby equipment and nursery items.

www.britishdoulas.co.uk (Tel: 020 7244 6053)
Provides information about hiring a doula.

About the Author

Clare Byam-Cook trained as a nurse at Westminster Hospital and qualified in 1976. After going on to do a midwifery course at Pembury Hospital in Kent and qualifying as a midwife in 1979, she then worked for four years at Queen Charlotte's Hospital in London until the birth of her first baby. In 1989 Clare was approached by ante-natal teacher Christine Hill to join Hill's Chiswick practice as her breast-feeding specialist and she has been there ever since.

During her years working with Christine Hill, Clare has gained invaluable experience in everything to do with breast-feeding, bottle-feeding, crying babies (and crying mothers!), and everything else associated with the day-to-day care of newborn babies. In addition to teaching at the ante-natal classes, she makes home visits to any mother who asks for her help, and says she has learnt more about babies and feeding problems from doing these home visits than in all her years spent working as a hospital midwife.

Clare has gained a reputation for being able to solve almost any breast-feeding problem and all her clients come to her by word-of-mouth referral from their friends, GPs, obstetricians, paediatricians, midwives and health visitors. Clare has never advertised her services and says that when the referrals dry up she knows it will be time for her to retire!

Clare feels that there is no better experience to be acquired than by being in a position to see the same problems time and time again. As a result, most of the advice she gives in this book is based on the knowledge she has gained during the many years she has been doing these home visits. It is not based solely on textbook theories.

Index